KU-334-584

J R Greenwood, R P C Morgan, J N Short
Bio-engineering: a field trial at Longham Wood Cutting, M20 Motorway
Construction Industry Research and Information Association
CIRIA Special Publication 128, 1996

ISBN 0 86017 458 1
© CIRIA 1996

Keywords		
Bio-engineering, slope stability, vegetation, Gault Clay		
Reader interest	**Classification**	
Civil engineers, geotechnical engineers, landscape architects	AVAILABILITY	Unrestricted
	CONTENT	Report of field trials
	STATUS	Committee Guided
	USER	Designers, specifiers and contractors for landscape works

Published by CIRIA, 6 Storey's Gate, Westminster, London SW1P 3AU. All rights reserved. No part of this publication may be reproduced or transmitted in any form or by any means, including photocopying and recording, without the written permission of the copyright holder, application for which should be addressed to the publisher. Such written permission must also be obtained before any part of this publication is stored in a retrieval system of any nature.

Foreword

The research leading to this report was carried out by the following, under contract to CIRIA, as research project *RP441: Field Test and Demonstration Site for Bio-Engineering*:

Mr J Greenwood	Symonds Travers Morgan, later Nottingham Trent University
Mr A Jones and Ms A Marsh	Symonds Travers Morgan
Mr N Coppin, Mr J Short and Mr M Webb	Wardell Armstrong
Professor R Morgan and Mr A Vickers	Silsoe College, Cranfield University

The project was guided by a Steering Group, and CIRIA and the research contractors wish to express their appreciation for the technical guidance and support given by the Group during the project and in reviewing the drafts of the report:

Mr F R D Chartres (Chairman)	Bullen & Partners *
Mr J Dowling	Balfour Beatty Civil Engineering Limited
Mr R Kent	L G Mouchel & Partners *
Mr I Richards	Richards Moorehead and Laing
Mr P Richardson	Symonds Travers Morgan
Mr R Snowdon	Transport Research Laboratory
Mr P Woodhead	DoE Construction Sponsorship Directorate

* as at 31 December 1995

CIRIA would also like to thank other individuals and organisations who have contributed to the technical discussion and assisted with the trials:

Mr J Baker	Union Railways
Mr D Barker	Geostructures Consulting
Mr A Baxter	Symonds Travers Morgan (M20 site)
Mr R Cooper	Symonds Travers Morgan
Mr J Connolly	Symonds Travers Morgan (M20 site)
Mr D Ivison	Highways Agency

CIRIA's Research Managers for this project were Mr D W Churcher and Mr G M Gray.

The project was funded by DoE Construction Sponsorship Directorate, Transport Research Laboratory on behalf of Road Engineering and Environmental Division, Highways Agency and received contributions-in-kind from the Highways Agency, Richards Moorehead and Laing and the research contractors listed above.

Contents

List of Figures

List of Tables

Plates

Glossary

Field capacity   The moisture content of the soil two or three days after having been saturated and after free drainage has practically ceased. Typical suctions at field capacity are between -5 and -10 kN/m^2.

Forbs   A generally non-woody, often flowering plant species usually associated with grass swards.

Matric potential   *See* **Water potential**.

Moisture content (gravimetric)   The amount of water contained in soil expressed by weight as a percentage of dry soil weight:

$$\text{Moisture content} = \frac{\text{Weight of water}}{\text{Weight of dry soil}} \times 100\%$$

Moisture content (volumetric)   Moisture content expressed in terms of volume:

$$\text{Volumetric moisture content} = \frac{\text{Volume of water}}{\text{Total volume of sample}} \times 100\%$$

The gravimetric and volumetric moisture contents are related by the following expression:

$$\text{Gravimetric moisture content} = \frac{\text{Volumetric moisture content}}{\text{Total volume of sample}}$$

Pore water pressure   Water pressure within the voids of the soil as might be measured by a standpipe or tensiometer device. Units are frequently head of water measured in metres (or sometimes cm) or the equivalent pressure in kilopascals (kPa), i.e. 1m head = 1 x γ_w = 10kN/m^2.

In some references, suction is recorded as pF units $\equiv \log_{10}$ (negative capillary suction head in cm).

γ_w represents the density of water.

Saturated soil   Soil with all the voids filled with water.

Soil suction   *See* Pore water pressure

Soil water pressure   *See* Pore water pressure

Water content   *See* Moisture content

Water potential   Relates the measured water pressure (h_w) to a hydraulic reference datum, such as the ground surface or the standing water table (h). This is illustrated as follows:

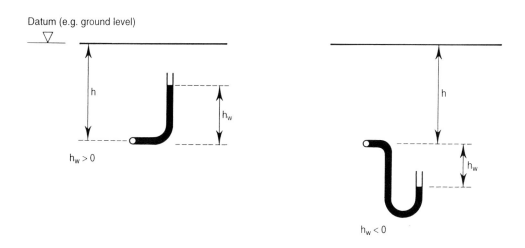

Datum (e.g. ground level)

Potential (relative to ground level) = $h_w - h$

1   Introduction

1.1   HISTORICAL DEVELOPMENT

The book 'Use of Vegetation in Civil Engineering' was published in 1990 as the outcome of a CIRIA research project aimed at providing technical guidance to practising engineers on the use of vegetation as an engineering material. To encourage the uptake of these promising techniques, CIRIA carried out an evaluation programme relating primarily to the use of vegetation in slope stabilisation by establishing trial demonstration sites in suitable locations.

The project 'Field evaluation and demonstration sites for bio-engineering' commenced with the research contractors Richards Moorehead and Laing, Silsoe College, Travers Morgan and Wardell Armstrong assessing sites which might be suitable for bio-engineering evaluation and demonstration purposes. A literature review and outline proposals for the establishment and monitoring of demonstration sites were prepared. Two possible sites, one in a cutting (Longham Wood Cutting) and one on an embankment, were found associated with the M20 motorway Junctions 5 to 8 improvement works at Maidstone, Kent.

Due to programming and budget restraints it was not possible to proceed with both sites but it was agreed by CIRIA, the Highways Agency, Department of Environment and supporting funders that the project should proceed on the site at Longham Wood Cutting.

The selected cutting was excavated in 1992 at a new cut slope as part of the M20 motorway Junctions 5 to 8 improvements. The cut slopes in this area have a history of shallow-seated slope failure.

Symonds Travers Morgan, Wardell Armstrong and Silsoe College have jointly carried out the research work, which included a programme of instrumentation and monitoring intended to demonstrate the potential value of vegetation to improve slope stability.

This report presents the details of the site, planting, instrumentation and monitoring over a two-year period. It summarises the results of the monitoring and discusses the conclusions to be drawn from them.

1.2   NATURE AND EXTENT OF THE ENGINEERING PROBLEM

Shallow-seated slope failures are defined for the purpose of this report as mass soil movements with a slip surface no more than 2 metres below the surface of the ground. The soil movement may be translational, rotational, or more commonly a combination of the two. Deep-seated failures are not considered since they are unlikely to be stabilised by vegetation.

Shallow-seated slope failures have occurred in many locations, particularly in the south and east of England, where naturally occurring, over-consolidated clays have been exposed in cuttings or re-used in embankments. A survey of motorway slopes was reported in 1985 (Parsons and Perry, 1985) where failures were recorded as a percentage of the total length of slope constructed of each soil material. Perry (1989) reported that out of 570km of motorway cuttings and embankment surveyed, 95% of the road slippages occurred within 1.5m of the surface (when measured vertically). Both cutting and embankment slopes excavated and constructed in Gault Clay had significantly higher failure rates (9.7% and 9.1% respectively) than any other geological stratum surveyed.

The A45 and M11 north of Cambridge have suffered over 30 embankment failures since their construction in the late 1970s (Johnson, 1985). These failures were typically shallow translational slides in the over-consolidated Gault Clay which was used to construct the embankments. Repair costs for excavation and granular replacement have been £10,000 – 15,000 per failure at 1980s prices (Greenwood, Holt and Herrick, 1985). Clearly, the cumulative cost of repairing such failures on a national scale is considerable and an understanding of the causes and possible means of prevention is highly desirable.

Engineering techniques are available for the repair and prevention of the shallow slips (Greenwood et al, 1985; Johnson, 1985) but the possible benefits available from selected planting regimes and vegetation management are less familiar to engineers.

1.3   REASONS FOR CHOOSING LONGHAM WOOD CUTTING

Longham Wood Cutting is a south facing cutting in Gault Clay located on the north side of the M20 motorway near Maidstone in Kent. The original cutting, built in 1960, at a slope of 1:3, had a history of shallow-seated slope failures associated with pre-existing failure planes within the Gault Clay.

As part of the M20 Junctions 5 to 8 improvements, it was required to widen the motorway at Longham Wood Cutting. The scheme was designed by Travers Morgan for the Highways Agency. Construction was carried out by Balfour Beatty, under the supervision of Travers Morgan.

Longham Wood Cutting was selected as a demonstration site for the following reasons:
- the cutting had a history of shallow-seated slope instability
- the cutting is in Gault Clay which has been reported as having high failure rates in cuttings and embankments
- the proposed timing for excavation was compatible with the research programme and funding
- the Contractor and supervisory staff would be available on site until 1995 to carry out planting, assist with site instrumentation, etc.
- the new cutting slope could be reprofiled to the steeper slopes required for the trial without endangering highway traffic.

1.4   RATIONALE

The objectives of the field evaluation and demonstration trials were twofold.
1. To provide a demonstration facility where the bio-engineering techniques could be seen in operation in order to encourage their wider adoption.
2. To provide an opportunity to compare different vegetation types and to gather field data on their relative performance and effects.

The vegetation is expected to strengthen the near-surface Gault Clay deposits in two principal ways.

1. It will reduce moisture content by evapotranspiration, hence increasing both the undrained shear strength and the effective stresses.

2. It will reinforce the mass structure of the fissured Gault Clay within the zone of root growth, by the direct effects of root tensile strength and soil binding.

The rationale behind the design of the trial site was influenced by both the practical limitation of site availability and the number of different treatments that could be considered within the available space. Layout was defined taking account of the following factors.

1. It is unlikely that the effects of the vegetation could be successfully monitored by direct observation of failures in the slope. Effects will therefore be assessed by monitoring the relevant factors that affect slope stability, i.e. moisture content and reinforcement.

2. The site is not set up as a fully replicated trial due to limitations of site area and resources. However, with the proposed treatment and monitoring regime, the site should generate useful data on the effects of vegetation.

3. Treatments are principally based on different vegetation types. The site was partially drained and on the secondary plots variable topsoil depths were placed to give additional treatment variation. Geotextile and vegetation combinations were not included as this would have increased the scale of the trial considerably. However, it would be of benefit to consider the use of geotextiles in future studies.

4. The minimum timescale for the influence of the vegetation to be effective would be about 5 years and the monitoring should continue for this period. If funds were available, it would be of benefit to extend this timescale.

2   Literature review

The full literature review carried out by Richards, Moorehead and Laing Ltd is included as Appendix A1. The salient points from this review are summarised below.

Greenwood et al (1985), drawing on the observations of Parsons and Perry (1985) and Farrar (1984, 1985), proposed the following mechanism for shallow failures on embankments within a few years of construction. When over-consolidated clay is excavated and placed on embankments, clay from the deeper horizons is frequently removed and used to form the surface material. This clay has the greatest suction as the greatest stress relief has taken place. Water from various sources, including rainfall and road drainage, steadily or seasonally reduces the suction, increases pore water pressure and lowers strength until failure occurs.

Various civil engineering methods of slope repair and strengthening are currently used. These include:

- granular replacement (Johnson, 1985; Greenwood et al, 1985) whereby the softened clay is removed and the profile reinstated with free-draining fill

- alternative construction methods (Johnson, 1985; Greenwood et al, 1985), for example lime addition, geogrid reinforcement, gabion walls

- surface stabilisation techniques using combinations of vegetation and geotextiles (Coppin and Richards, 1990; Barker, 1986).

Vegetation can aid the stabilisation of shallow failure planes in clay slopes by:

- removing soil water and intercepting some rainfall for direct re-evaporation (Gray, 1978)

- increasing shear strength, as demonstrated in the review by Coppin and Richards (1990) in which a simplified model is presented for analysing the contribution of root tensile strength

- roots of more than 20mm diameter acting as individual soil anchors (Coppin and Richards, 1990)

- vegetation cover which shades the surface from baking by the sun and provides a root network which restrains severe cracking of the soil (Coppin and Richards, 1990)

- combining bio-engineering techniques with inert materials.

Vegetation species selected for stabilising slopes should satisfy the following characteristics:

- rapid transpiration, winter transpiration activity and an extensive root system, all of which will contribute to the removal of soil water

- rapid deep (>1.5m) root growth to strengthen the failure plane

- high leaf area ratios with persistence during hot summer periods to produce surface shading.

Often a mixture of species of trees, shrubs and ground vegetation will be necessary to satisfy these requirements.

The understanding of slope failure and the performance of various types of vegetation would be greatly enhanced from a programme of field trials in which changes in soil and plant parameters are continuously monitored.

The literature review endorsed the need for the field trial study and concluded that the lack of practical research on techniques for the stabilisation of clay slopes prone to shallow failure could be seen both from the extent of the problem and the lack of trials experience. Particular aspects worthy of study were considered to be:

- the modification of soil moisture regimes by various types of vegetation, including herbaceous ground cover, shrubs and trees

- methods and species capable of rooting through the potential failure plane to strengthen this soil horizon, before soil re-wetting reaches critical limits

- the value of geotextiles, particularly in constructed embankments, as deeply buried 'envelopes' to restrain softened soils.

A trial set up in an area known to be prone to slope failure could provide valuable data for use in future slope design, and act as a demonstration of the validity of bio-engineering techniques for such applications.

3   Longham Wood Cutting

3.1   SITE DESCRIPTION AND HISTORY

Longham Wood Cutting is located to the north of the M20 motorway, adjacent to the eastbound carriageway, between Junctions 7 and 8. A site location plan is given in Figure 3.1.

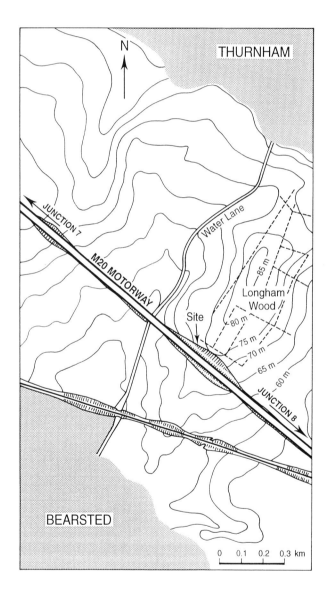

Figure 3.1 Site location plan

In 1989 Travers Morgan identified several slips which had occurred in the cutting at various times. These are summarised in Table 3.1.

A history of remedial works undertaken at the site is given in Table 3.2.

Table 3.1 History of failures in Longham Wood Cutting

Cutting	Date	Comments[1]
Longham Wood North[3]	1960	Slope constructed at 1:3
	1968	Local failure in east end
	1970	Additional slips
	1972	Additional slips
	1976	Major slips in March 1975
		Remedial works in north slopes in 1976
	1981	No signs of further movement
	1983	No signs of further movement in reinstatement. Area to east of reinstatement shows recent slips below berm
	1992	Slope cut back at 1 in 6 for widening associated with M20 improvements
	1993	Trial site prepared at 1 in 3 slope
Longham Wood South [2, 3]	1976	Shallow slips and minor bulging in localised areas at eastern end
	1981	Shallow slips at chainage 62,900 but backscar covered in vegetation
	1983	Some bulging and general unevenness with slip and bulging at chainage 62,900 areas
	1992	Slope not affected by M20 improvements

Notes:

1. Table prepared by Travers Morgan (1989).
2. No data given for Longham Wood South prior to 1976.
3. The maximum depth of the North cutting is 17m below original ground level and of the South cutting is 5.0m.

Table 3.2 Remedial works undertaken at Longham Wood Cutting

Contract Chainage	Treatment	Comments[1]
North Side		
Extent not reported, see below	Failed 'mantle' removed and replaced with 2–3 metres of 'free-draining' shingle	Undertaken by Kent County Council in 1976
9185 – 9245	Counterfort drains installed (10 metre centres, 3m deep)	1985 Maintenance Contract
9245 – 9515	Approximately 500mm thickness of 'free-draining' shingle removed as a result of regrading	1985 Maintenance Contract
9515 – 9570	Ballast replacement	1985 Maintenance Contract
9570 – 9605	Counterfort drains installed (10 metre centres, 3m deep)	1985 Maintenance Contract
South Side		
9175 – 9250	Counterfort drains installed (10 metre centres, 3m deep)	1985 Maintenance Contract
9250 – 9345	Ballast replacement	1985 Maintenance Contract
9345 – 9605	Counterfort drains installed (10 metre centres, 3m deep)	1985 Maintenance Contract

Note:

1. Table prepared by Travers Morgan (1989).

GEOLOGICAL AND GEOTECHNICAL INFORMATION

The geological units encountered in the cutting were described by Travers Morgan in 1989. The system of subdivisions of the Gault Clay is given below in Table 3.3, starting with the youngest stratum. Figure 3.2 is a section through the cutting showing the subdivisions.

Table 3.3 Subdivisions of Gault Clay

Unit	Description[1]
Solifluxion[2] deposits	Consists of remoulded Gault Clay with chalk pellets, tufa nodules and flint fragments. Shear surfaces or zones present, usually at base. Generally 1–3m thick.
Cryoturbated[3] Gault Clay	Shear planes are randomly orientated and relatively steeply inclined. Fissuring occurs at spacing <25mm with irregular orientation. Sometimes absent, rarely extends below 6m from ground surface.
Weathered Gault Clay	Chemical weathering results in brown grey colour. Fissuring is regular and occurs at spacing 50 – 100mm. Typically extends to 9m below ground surface.
Unweathered Gault Clay	Stiff fissured dark grey plastic clay which is stiffer than weathered Gault Clay. Fissuring occurs at spacing 100mm. Most fissures are matt and planar.

Notes:

1. Table prepared by Travers Morgan in 1989.

2. Solifluxion is the downslope movement of material.

3. Cryoturbation is disturbance by frost churning (periglacial origin).

Norwest Holst Soil Engineering Ltd carried out a site investigation in 1988 under the supervision of Travers Morgan for the Department of Transport. Two exploratory boreholes E55 and E56 were sunk in the vicinity of the cutting as part of this investigation and are indicated on Figure 3.2. A summary of the test results is given below in Table 3.4.

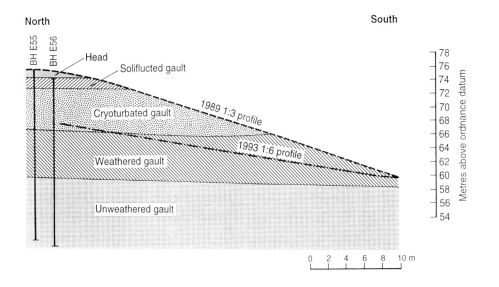

Figure 3.2 Section through Longham Wood Cutting

Table 3.4 Summary of test results of Gault Clay

Test parameter	Result	Comments
Moisture content	20–29%	Moisture contents of all samples in investigation were reported to be 5–10% higher than plastic limits for samples within 5m depth.
Liquid limit	59–81%	
Plastic limit	19–27%	Most samples tested in investigation were reported to have very high plasticity.
Undrained shear strength	Above 60kN/m² below 3.5m depth. Above 100kN/m² below 8.0m depth.	Fissures may influence shear strength. Tests not carried out on samples from Longham Wood Cutting.
Coefficient of volume compressibility	0.05–0.55m²/mN within 0–10m depth. 0.05–0.10m²/mN below 10m depth.	Tests not carried out on samples from Longham Wood Cutting.
Coefficient of consolidation	0.4–5.5m²/yr within 0-10m depth 0.5–2.5m²/yr below 10m depth	Tests not carried out on samples from Longham Wood Cutting.
Shear strength parameter from triaxial tests	$c' = 12$kN/m², $\varnothing' = 23°$	Drained triaxial tests were carried out on samples from Longham Wood Cutting. Obtained by linear regression of all triaxial tests.
	$c' = 7$kN/m², $\varnothing' = 26°$	Peak strength parameters for effective stress levels < 150kN/m².
Shear strength parameters from shear box tests	$\varnothing'_r = 16°$	Shear box tests were carried out on samples from Longham Wood Cutting. Normal stress <50kN/m² $\varnothing'_r$ is reduced at higher stress levels.
Dry density	$\gamma = 1.48$Mg/m³	Average figure from test results.

Note:

1. Samples are from Longham Wood Cutting unless stated otherwise in the Comments column above.

4 Site preparation and plot establishment

4.1 ORIGINAL AND AMENDED SLOPE DESIGNS

The slope of the original cutting was approximately 1:3. As part of the improvements to the motorway, the new slope was excavated at a cut angle of 1:6. At an angle of 1:6 the risk of a shallow failure is low and the slope for the primary trial plots was increased to the original slope of 1:3. This increased the risk of instability and gave a greater potential for the effects of vegetation to be demonstrated. Motorway traffic was protected from any shallow failures by a near horizontal berm between the 1:3 slope and the carriageway. The original and amended profiles are shown in Figure 4.1.

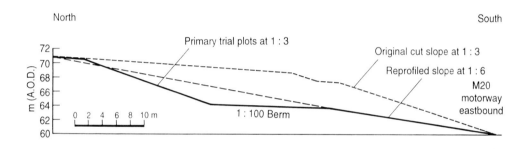

Figure 4.1 Section through the demonstration site

4.2 PREPARATION OF THE DEMONSTRATION SITE

The demonstration site was split into two sections comprising western 'primary' trial plots at 1:3 and eastern 'secondary' trial plots at 1:6. This is shown in Figure 4.2.

At the base of the 1:3 slope is a near horizontal berm, which provides access and a safety area should there be any slippage of the slope. The primary plots are shown in Plate 1, looking east to west.

Counterfort drains 6m deep have been installed where indicated in Figure 4.2 at 10m spacings and were filled with free draining material. The purpose of these drains was to maintain a low groundwater level in the slope, and thus reduce the potential pore water pressure and increase the stability. These counterfort drains are present over the eastern section of the primary plots and over all of the secondary plots.

A conventional french drain was constructed along the top of the cutting as part of the M20 improvement contract. Its purpose is to collect surface water from the adjacent farmland and to intercept water from existing agricultural drains cut by the construction of the new highway slope.

The secondary trial plots of the site comprise an area of 21 plots, each 10m square, in a 3 x 7 array.

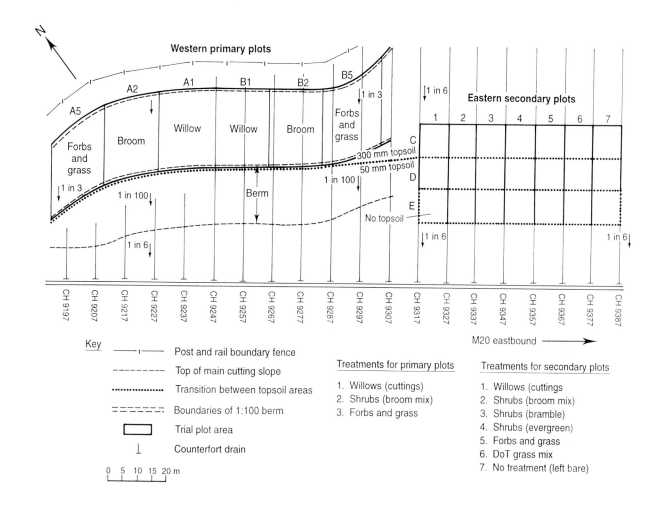

Key

— · — Post and rail boundary fence

- - - - - - Top of main cutting slope

·············· Transition between topsoil areas

= = = = = Boundaries of 1:100 berm

☐ Trial plot area

⊥ Counterfort drain

0 5 10 15 20 m

Treatments for primary plots

1. Willows (cuttings)
2. Shrubs (broom mix)
3. Forbs and grass

Treatments for secondary plots

1. Willows (cuttings
2. Shrubs (broom mix)
3. Shrubs (bramble)
4. Shrubs (evergreen)
5. Forbs and grass
6. DoT grass mix
7. No treatment (left bare)

Figure 4.2 Plan of bio-engineering demonstration site at Longham Wood Cutting

The primary plots were topsoiled between 24 October 1993 and 4 November 1993. Prior to topsoil spreading the surface of the Gault Clay was cultivated. Soils were placed to their full depth of 300mm in one operation. The placement method used was to free tip and blade down slope using a CAT D6 dozer. During placement the weather was cool and overcast but dry.

The topsoil was placed on the secondary plots on two occasions. The first occasion was between 21 June 1993 and 1 July 1993 and the weather was hot, sunny and dry. The machine used was a scraper box and tractor unit. The topsoil was placed to 300mm during this first occasion and 'cut' down to the correct thickness during the second occasion, which was between 22 October 1993 and 23 October 1993 when the weather was cool, cloudy and rainy. The different topsoil thicknesses of 300mm, 50mm and nil are shown on Figure 4.2. The machine used was a Komatsu D6 track dozer along with a Komatsu PC210 track excavator.

On all plots the Gault Clay surface was moist and the placed soils were moist and plastic at the time of placement.

These site conditions were not ideal and the placement of moist soils can lead to problems of smeared and compacted layers. Such layers may restrict root development and influence the potential of the vegetation.

4.3   **GEOTECHNICAL REGIMES AND VEGETATION TYPES**

Within the primary and secondary plots, five different geotechnical regimes and seven different vegetation types have been used. Each different plot on the site is referenced by a unique combination of geotechnical regime (a letter from A to E) and a vegetation type (number from 1 to 7), e.g. plot B2 has 300mm topsoil, is drained on a 1:3 slope and is planted with broom mix shrubs. The ranges of geotechnical regimes and vegetation types are described below:

Geotechnical regimes

A.   300mm topsoil, undrained, 1:3 slope
B.   300mm topsoil, drained, 1:3 slope
C.   300mm topsoil, drained, 1:6 slope
D.   50mm topsoil, drained, 1:6 slope
E.   No topsoil, drained, 1:6 slope

Vegetation Types

1.   Willows/Alders
2.   Shrubs (broom mix)
3.   Shrubs (bramble)
4.   Shrubs (evergreen)
5.   Forbs and grass
6.   Department of Transport grass mix
7.   None – left bare

Treatments 6 and 7 were included to provide a control treatment. Details of actual species used are given in the Specification for the trial areas, included as Appendix A2.

The primary plots were used to test regimes A and B, each with vegetation types 1, 2 and 5. The secondary plots combined regimes C, D and E with all vegetation types (1 to 7).

4.4   **PLOT ESTABLISHMENT**

Cultivation and planting/sowing operations on site were delayed due to both contractual arrangements and the very wet spring of 1994. Plots were sprayed and cultivated in mid-April 1994 with all plots except plot 4 being planted or sown by 4 May 1994. Evergreen shrubs were planted in plot 4 by 11 May 1994.

All planting was either as pot grown stock or, in the case of the willows, peat plugs. Due to the delayed planting, the bare root stock, as specified, was not available.

Four different fertilisation treatments were applied to the plots and they are summarised in Table 4.1.

Plots with topsoil thicknesses of 300mm (A, B and C) were cultivated to 225mm then rotovated to 150mm depth (agreed amendment to Specification). Plots with topsoil thicknesses of 50mm and zero (D and E) were cultivated to a depth of 50mm.

Table 4.1 Summary of fertilisation treatments

Geotechnical regime	Vegetation Type						
	1	**2**	**3**	**4**	**5**	**6**	**7**
A	i	i	N/A	N/A	ii	N/A	N/A
B	i	i	N/A	N/A	ii	N/A	N/A
C	i	i	i	i	ii	i	iv
D	i	i	i	i	ii	i	iv
E	iii	iii	iii	iii	iii	iii	iv

Key:

Treatment	Details
i	10:20:20 Compound fertiliser at a rate of 40g/m² (proportions are agreed amendment to Specification) 0:22:0 Superphosphate at a rate of 25g/m²
ii	0:20:30 Compound fertiliser at a rate of 40g/m² (proportions are agreed amendment to Specification) 0:22:0 Superphosphate at a rate of 25g/m²
iii	10:20:20 Compound fertiliser at a rate of 80g/m²
iv	No fertiliser application
N/A	This combination of geotechnical regime and vegetation type was not included in the field trial
Note:	ratios are the proportions of nitrogen, phosphate and potash ($N:P_2O_5:K_2O$) respectively.

Surface cultivation was effective to a depth of 75 – 100mm, leaving a medium to coarse tilth. At the time of a site visit on 5 May 1994, occasional weed growth was evident in some plots. This had survived both the spraying and the cultivation. Surface soils were very dry at the time of the site visit. Deeper soils below approximately 150mm and the surface of the clay cutting below the placed soils were moist.

The late season planting and sowing of the plots increased the risk of vegetation failure due to the plants' vulnerability to summer drought. The degree of failure is partially dependent on the weather conditions over the months following planting. Although the 1994 summer was relatively dry, the use of container-grown stock and peat plugs helped to increase the chances of survival.

4.5 MAINTENANCE STRATEGY

The proposed management strategy for the different vegetation types and soil cover regimes were as follows:

- willows are to be coppiced at regular intervals once fully established. The cycle time will be a function of how well they put on growth but is likely to be every 6 to 8 years. Willow stems were cut following planting to encourage multiple shoot growth

- shrub and evergreen plots are only to be cut back as part of general maintenance to ensure good health and growth

- grass and forb plots are to be cut only once per year after all flowering plants have set seed in the autumn. This was carried out in September 1994 and 1995

- DTp grass mix plots are to be cut twice per year in spring and autumn. In the first year these plots were cut three times to promote tillering and aid good establishment. The plots were cut twice in 1995

- bare ground plots are to be sprayed off to maintain them in a vegetation free state

- the non-topsoiled plots will have a lower fertility than the other areas. As such it is intended to apply supplementary fertiliser in the second full year of growth (1996)
- to ensure full establishment of all plots, any plant failures are to be replaced. There were considerable losses during the summer droughts of 1995 which required replanting of much of the evergreen (plot 4) and bramble (plot 3) shrubs.

A more detailed description of both the establishment and maintenance requirements of each plot is given in Appendix A2.

5   Instrumentation and monitoring

5.1   INTRODUCTION

Scientific monitoring was concentrated on the six primary plots. A limited programme of data collection and observation was carried out on the 21 secondary plots.

The specific objective of the scientific monitoring was to show whether vegetation treatments had a significant effect on the stability of the slope and, if so, the time taken to achieve that effect.

Since it was not possible to monitor slope failure directly, the monitoring strategy was to measure the changes taking place in the geotechnical properties of the soil material. The data was analysed to gain an understanding of the processes which operated at the site and to evaluate and quantify the effects of the different bio-engineering treatments.

5.2   MONITORING PROGRAMME

The monitoring programme focused on three aspects:

- vegetation growth and root distribution
- changes in soil moisture content and soil pore water pressures and suctions
- soil strength, as modified over time by weathering and root reinforcement.

Information about the instruments installed is given in Table 5.1, and a plan of the locations of the instruments in the primary plots is shown in Figure 5.1. Figure 5.2 shows the instrumentation and testing locations relative to each neutron probe access tube. Neutron probe access tubes were installed in the centre of each secondary plot.

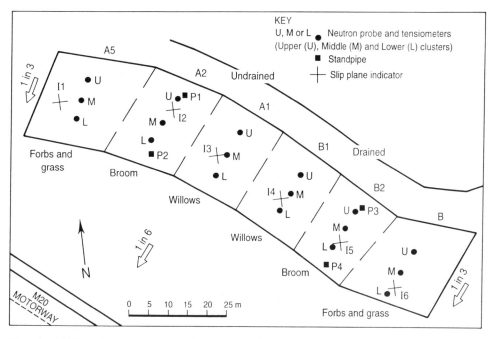

Figure 5.1 Plan of instrumentation in the primary plots

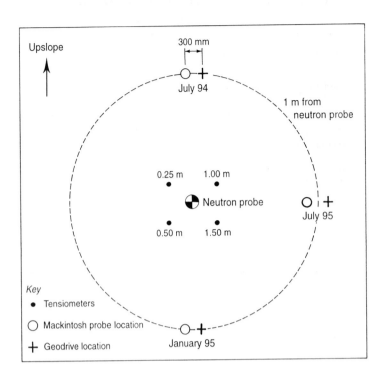

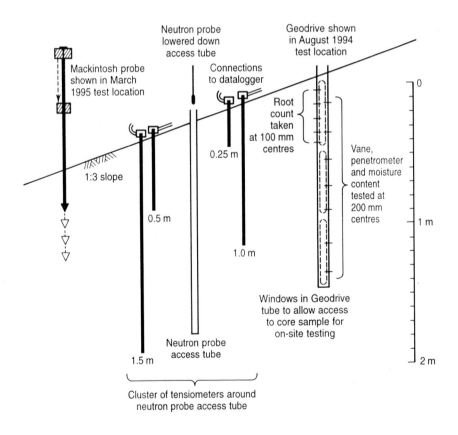

Figure 5.2 Plan and section of each instrumentation cluster around a neutron probe
access tube

Most of the monitoring was discontinuous with measurements made on a regular basis to give 'snap shot' indications of the differences between the treatments. Timing varied depending on the measurement being made (Table 5.2). For example, soil moisture content was measured monthly using the neutron probes whereas vegetation characteristics were recorded annually.

Table 5.1 Instrumentation installed

Instrument	Number	Locations	Date installed/ Installer
Standpipe piezometer	4	Plots A2 and B2	November 1993/ Balfour Beatty
Slip plane indicator	6	Centre of each primary plot	November 1993/ Balfour Beatty
Neutron probe access tube	18 + 21	3 per primary plot and 1 per secondary plot	April 1994/ Silsoe College
Tensiometer	72	4 depths per location, 3 locations per primary plot	As above

Table 5.2 Monitoring regime

Instrument	Number	Locations	Dates read/ Reader
Standpipe piezometer	4	Plots A2 and B2	Monthly from June 1994 to August 1995/ Travers Morgan
Slip plane indicator	6	Centre of each primary plot	As above
Neutron probe	18 + 21	3 per primary plot and 1 per secondary plot	Regularly (approx. 6 weekly) from July 1994/ Silsoe College
Tensiometer	72	4 depths per location, 3 locations per primary plot	July 1994 then continuously, i.e. 6 times daily, between October 1994 and August 1995/ Silsoe College
Mackintosh probe	18	3 per primary plot	August 1994, March 1995, August 1995/ Travers Morgan
Core samples	18	3 per primary plot to 1.5m depth	As above
Moisture content[1]		0.2m centres from each core sample	As above
Shear strength by hand vane and pocket penetrometer[1]		As above	As above
Root content[1]		Counted at every 100mm depth in core sample	Sample obtained by Travers Morgan, counted by Wardell Armstrong
Top growth	6 + 21	Each primary plot and secondary plot	August 1994, August 1995/ Wardell Armstrong
Photographs		Each plot and whole site	August 1994, March 1995, August 1995

Notes
1. Tests carried out on core samples.

Continuous monitoring of soil suction was undertaken, with 4-hourly readings stored in dataloggers and downloaded at monthly intervals. Further details of the monitoring carried out are given in sections 5.3, 5.4 and 5.5.

Plate 5 shows an instrumentation cluster with a neutron probe access tube surrounded by four tensiometers wired up to a datalogger.

5.3   VEGETATION MONITORING

5.3.1   Top growth

Top growth was recorded in each primary and secondary plot once per year, using 3 quadrats per plot. These were specific areas of each plot within which vegetation was monitored. Quadrats were recorded for cover/abundance of each species using the *Domin* scale, together with the overall height, vigour and density of the vegetation cover. The *Domin* scale utilises a score of 1 to 10 for percentage degree of cover of vegetation as shown in Table 5.3.

Table 5.3 The Domin Scale

Score	Percentage Cover
1	Few individuals <4% cover
2	Several individuals <4% cover
3	Many individuals <4% cover
4	4% – 10% cover
5	11% – 25% cover
6	26% – 33% cover
7	34% – 50% cover
8	51% – 75% cover
9	76% – 91% cover
10	91% – 100% cover

5.3.2   Root growth

The root growth was assessed by breaking the cores taken for geotechnical monitoring at 100mm intervals down the soil profile and counting the number of roots at the break point. Unfortunately the core tubes used did not allow the soil core to be removed and all analysis was carried out through a window in the side of the casing, which proved difficult. The diameter of the core sampler used was noted in each case and the root count normalised to an 80mm diameter sample.

5.4   HYDROLOGICAL MONITORING

The following hydrological instruments were used:

5.4.1   Neutron probe

The purpose of the neutron probe was to measure moisture content, which can be related to both soil suction and pore pressure (up to saturation). The probes can only give 'snapshot' readings hence regular readings were required.

The probe was lowered down 50mm diameter, 1.5m long aluminium access tubes which were installed permanently in the ground. The access tubes were installed on site using a 50 mm geodrive drilling rig. Care was taken to ensure good contact between the soil and the sides of the access tube. During installation, strenuous efforts were made to minimise poor contact. Any gaps between the soil and the access tubes were filled with soil arisings (Gault Clay).

The neutron probe contains a radioactive source emitting fast neutrons which are slowed down (thermalised) by hydrogen ions in the soil. The thermalised or slow neutrons are then counted by a detector also housed in the probe. Since most soil hydrogen ions are present in the soil water, the concentration of thermalised neutrons can be related to the volumetric soil water content. The values apply to a 40 – 50cm diameter sphere around the position of the neutron probe. Correct use of the neutron probe requires careful calibration for each soil type using gravimetric measurements of soil moisture content.

5.4.2 Tensiometers

Tensiometers, along with their associate transducers, wiring and dataloggers, were used to measure soil suction and to calculate from this moisture content and moisture flux.

The tensiometer is a hollow porous ceramic probe which is filled with water to exclude air. When buried in the soil, water moves freely between the soil and the probe so that the water in the probe attains an equilibrium with the soil water. As the soil dries out water flows out of the probe and develops an increased suction; water flows into the probe as the soil wets up and the suction decreases. The negative pressure or suction is measured automatically by using flexible tubing to connect the probe to a vacuum gauge or a pressure transducer. The transducer is connected in turn to a data logger to record the reading every 4 hours, although it can also be read manually.

To work properly, the tensiometer must have good contact with the soil and the instrument must be kept filled with water. The measurement fails when the soil water tension exceeds about 0.8 bar (80 kPa), beyond which bubbles of air accumulate inside the ceramic probe, expanding as the pressure falls and cutting the hydraulic contact. The tensiometer then has to be recharged with water before further measurements can be made.

If a calibration is obtained for the soil between tension and soil moisture content, the measurements can be used to provide an estimate of soil moisture content.

The tensiometers were gently pushed into the bases of 25 mm diameter screw auger holes at depths of 0.25m, 0.5m 1.0m and 1.5m.

5.4.3 Rainfall data

The rain gauge installed at the M20 Improvements site offices was used to provide rainfall data for the early monitoring period. This was correlated to rainfall data from the meteorological office at Boxley so that this source could be used in the later stages of the monitoring after the site office rain gauge had been removed. Site rainfall was recorded on normal workings days only so that the first reading after a weekend or holiday period is the cumulative total rainfall since the previous reading. The anomalies between the meteorological office readings and the site readings are due to the recording regime used on site.

5.5 GEOTECHNICAL MONITORING

The following geotechnical instruments were installed or tests were carried out:

5.5.1 Standpipes

The standpipes were installed by Balfour Beatty in November 1993, located as shown in Figure 5.1 and positioned to a depth of 2.9m to measure groundwater levels in the cutting. The standpipe comprised a 50mm diameter scaffold tube which was perforated with 5mm diameter holes and wrapped in Terram 1000 over the bottom 1m. It was installed in a 100mm diameter augured hole and the annulus between tube and hole was backfilled with a sand filter over the bottom 1m length. The remainder was backfilled with clay arisings. The tops of the standpipe tubes projected approximately 0.3m above the ground and were covered with endcaps. The standpipes were read by a simple dip-meter.

5.5.2 Slip plane indicators

Slip plane indicators were installed by Balfour Beatty in November 1993 comprising 25mm diameter PVC flexible tubes positioned to 3m depth in 75mm diameter holes. The annuli were backfilled with sand up to 0.5m below ground level and then clay. They were read with a plumb rod. Resistance to lowering or raising the plumb rod would be indicative of ground movement affecting the verticality of the tube.

5.5.3 Mackintosh probes

The purpose of Mackintosh probing was to give an indication of the strength of the Gault Clay. The apparatus consists of a rod with a 25mm diameter cone whose base is of slightly larger diameter than the rod. The cone was driven into the ground by a 4kg hammer which was allowed to fall 400mm. The test recorded the number of blows of the hammer for the cone to penetrate the ground in 100mm increments over the specified depth (2.0m).

5.5.4 Core samples

Core samples were taken at a distance of 1m from the neutron probes in the primary plots. Geodrive sampling equipment of 60mm or 76mm diameter was used. Initial attempts to incorporate a transparent plastic liner were not successful. Hand vane tests and pocket penetrometer tests were carried out at approximately 200mm intervals on the geodrive samples. Root count tests were also performed. Samples were taken approximately every 200mm for later moisture content determination. The geodrive holes were backfilled and surface sealed with arisings. Plates 2 and 4 show geodrive sampling on the primary plots. Plate 3 shows an extracted sample being analysed for root count. Plate 6 shows hand vane tests being carried out on a core sample.

6   Results and discussion

6.1   VEGETATION RESULTS

6.1.1   General observations

The plots, having been established in winter 1993 spring 1994, were last monitored in
August 1995, monitoring being carried out as per the schedule presented in Section 5.5.
Within this short time-span full establishment of the vegetation would not be expected,
particularly on the plots planted with tree and shrub species. It is also of note that the
plots have undergone varying extremes of weather with a very wet winter (1994/95)
followed by an exceptionally hot, dry summer (1995).

Despite these factors most plots have populations of the planted/sown species and losses
tend to be centred on the 'no topsoil' secondary plots. Invasion of non-sown species had
been a problem and the current standard maintenance regime has only partially
overcome this. Additional works to control invasive weeds have been specified for
future maintenance.

Some damage to vegetation has been caused by trampling around the instrumentation
areas during monitoring. This relates to both the regular hydrological monitoring and
the two geotechnical/root monitoring sessions. Problems are particularly acute during
the winter period when soils are wet. Procedures are being adopted to minimise this
effect but some disturbance is inevitable.

Differences between drained and undrained plots are not obviously apparent in the
vegetation growth at this stage of the plants' development. Establishment has been
similar in both drained and undrained areas although the 1:3 slope will have provided
sufficient surface drainage to ensure that the upper soil layer did not become saturated.
As such, significant differences in establishment would not be expected. However,
future growth rates may be influenced by this factor.

6.1.2   Surface vegetation

The full results of the first two years monitoring of the surface vegetation are presented
as tables in the Data Appendix available from CIRIA as a separate document. These set
out the information in terms of the planted and non-planted species, the results being
expressed as domin values (see Section 5.3.1). General descriptions of each treatment
are presented within this section.

Willows and alders

On the main plots establishment has been successful with very few failures. The
different varieties have different growth habit but most plants are 1.5 to 2m tall. The
shorter growing cultivars, at 1 to 1.5m, tend to be very bushy in structure so putting on a
similar volume of growth to the taller plants. By August 95 ground cover by the willows
was approximately 30%.

On the deep topsoiled secondary plots the growth is similar to that of the main plots.
Growth on the 150m topsoil plot is consistent across the area but less vigorous, most

plants being less than 1m in height. On the plots without topsoil growth is poor, up to only 50cm in height and plants were suffering from the summer drought, this including some plant failure.

Broom and gorse

The establishment of these species from seed, the technique used on these plots, is likely to take 2 to 3 years. The lupin was included in the mix as this should establish more quickly providing an early cover. However, in the conditions encountered on these plots establishment may be delayed as the clays are not an ideal soil type for broom and gorse.

In all plots the sown species are found only sporadically across the area (<5%), however those plants present are up to 30cm in height and some of the lupin have flowered. The sown species are invasive by nature so although populations are low at present it is likely that they will eventually dominate the plots. The secondary plot growth is similar to that of the main plots, except on the non-topsoiled area where growth is weak and some die, back was evident.

The plots do have a high cover of colonising species of both grasses and forbs which will affect growth of the sown species. However in the first year of growth some vegetative cover is required to protect what would otherwise be large areas of bare ground. The need for weed control will be considered in years 3 and 4.

Grass and forb mix

On the main plots both sown grass and forb species have established well and have developed a 50 – 60% ground cover. The only sown species not found on the plots are the field scabious and white campion (see section A2.4.5 for the full list).

Non-sown species are also common with possible domination by such plants as bristly ox-tongue and creeping thistle if not controlled. The practicality of species-specific weed control, although possible on the plots, must be considered in terms of full-scale usage of such a treatment. It may be more realistic to accept some level of invasion of non-sown species as representing a 'real' situation.

As in all other vegetation types growth is less vigorous on the non-topsoiled secondary plots where considerable areas of bare ground are present.

Bramble mix

This mix is only planted on the secondary plots. On the 300mm topsoil, plot growth is healthy for both the rosa and bramble varieties. However after only 18 months growth, ground cover is low at approximately 10 – 15% and areas of grass and forb invasion have required control by spraying.

On the shallow topsoils growth is consistent but less vigorous and on the non-topsoiled areas the plants looked stressed with sign of some die-back.

Evergreen shrubs

These plots, again only established on the secondary area, have suffered badly from the 1995 summer drought. Having established well in 1994, considerable die-back and plant loss has occurred over the last year. The periwinkle has survived the best, the laurel and cotoneaster showing significant die-back. Dense weed growth on the 300mm topsoil plots has not been effectively controlled by spraying and will have contributed to the decline in the condition of the planted shrubs. On the non-top soiled plots no laurel has survived and the condition of the other plants is poor.

DoT grass mix

On the 300mm topsoil plot, establishment is good with high ground cover and high populations (approximately 30% cover) of the sown species. This cover is, however, dominated by white clover. Weed invasion is again common on all plots. Ground cover on the 150 mm topsoils areas is similar to that on the deeper soils. However on the bare subsoil plots cover of sown species is only some 5 – 10% and large cracks in the soil have appeared. On this plot bare ground is over 50% and plants had die back due to the summer drought.

6.1.3   Root growth

The patterns of root growth on the main plots are shown in Figures 6.1 and 6.2. These are for each of the main plots and the data used are averages of the three replicates taken in each treatment. The monitoring method used is described in Section 5.3. As, would be expected these data show a general increase in both the number of roots, and the depth of roots, with time. By August 1995 maximum root depth was 45cm.

The pie chart representations in Figure 6.2 are designed to illustrate the overall distribution of roots with depth for each treatment at August 1995. The most obvious factor here is that over 75% of all rooting is still within 150mm of the soil surface, and as such will have very little effect on the geotechnical characteristics of the slope at this stage.

No detailed analysis of rooting patterns is possible at this point due to the high percentage of non-sown species present on all plots and the early stages of development of most vegetation types. With time, more distinct patterns should develop. Also no measurement of root diameter has been made as most roots are fibrous, acting to extract moisture from the soil but adding little tensile strength. As plants develop, particularly the willows and wood shrubs, tensile strength will be taken into account during the monitoring.

The use of three replicates to measure root density is too few to provide statistically valid results due the very high degree of variability present in natural systems. However the method employed will give an indication of the rooting pattern from which broad conclusions can be drawn on the effects identified by the hydrological and geotechnical monitoring.

6.2   HYDROLOGICAL RESULTS

6.2.1   Tensiometer data

Results for the plots are available for the following periods:

A1, A2 and A5	B1, B2 and B5
19 October 1994 – 1 December 1994	19 October 1994 – 1 December 1994
7 January 1995 – 14 January 1995	21 January 1995 – 10 August 1995
27 April 1995 – 16 May 1995	
1 July 1995 – 7 July 1995	

GRASS AND FORBS

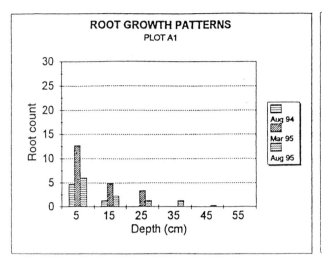

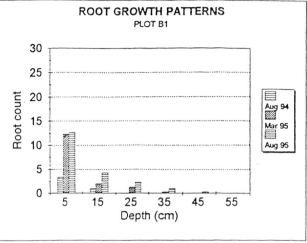

BROOM AND GORSE

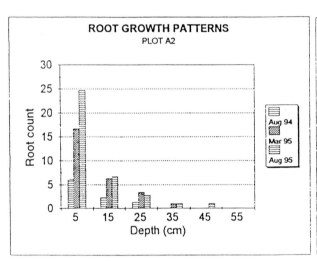

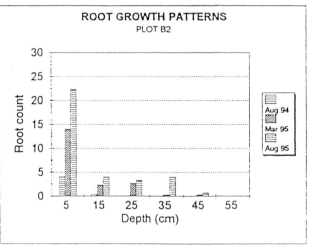

WILLOWS

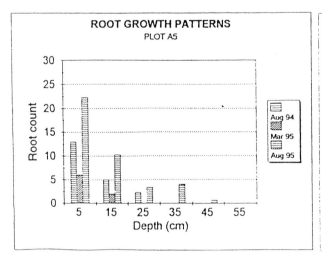

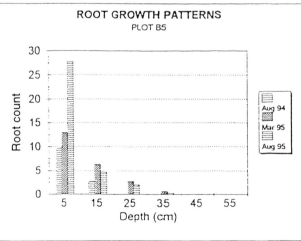

Figure 6.1 Root growth patterns, August 1994 – August 1995

GRASS AND FORBS

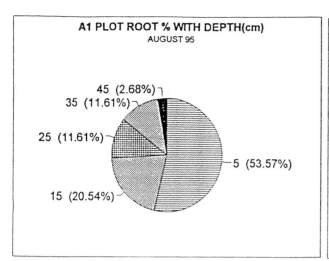

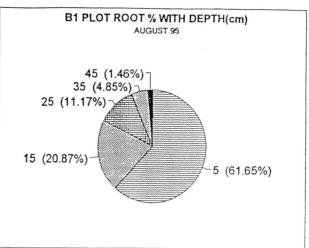

BROOM AND GORSE

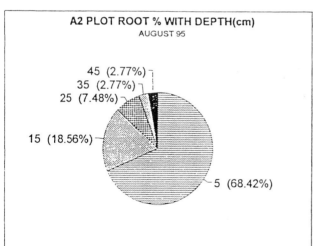

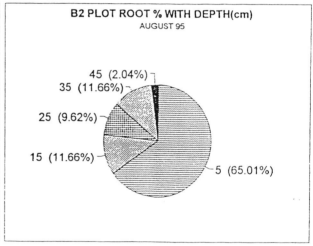

WILLOWS

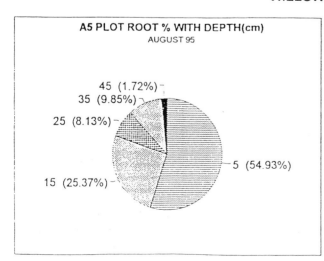

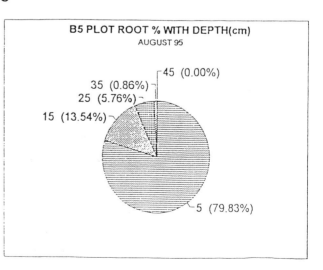

Figure 6.2 Percentage distribution of roots with depth at August 1995

The incomplete data set for the A plots is due to a variety of problems, initially with the data logger programme, then site damage and also earth loops in the wiring causing signal noise and power drainage.

From analysis of the data there are as yet no clear differences between treatments, and no differences that may indicate a response to vegetation growth over time. Therefore some general observations are presented to illustrate the type and implications of the data collected.

Figures 6.3 and 6.4 show daily midday tensiometer readings for the middle instrument nests for plots A1 and B2 for the period 19 October 1994 to 1 December 1994. These are typical of data sets for all the plots over the winter months.

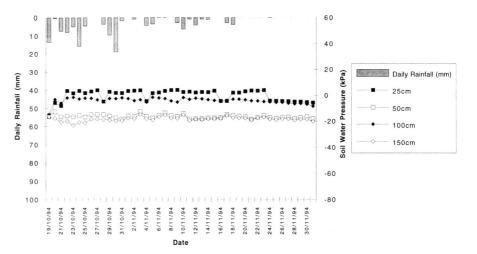

Figure 6.3 Midday tensiometer data for Plot A1 (middle)

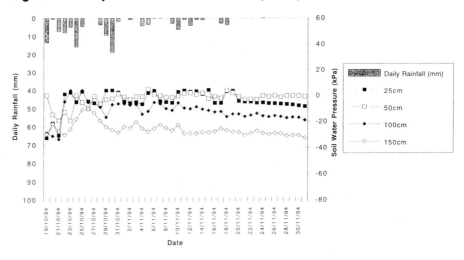

Figure 6.4 Midday tensiometer data for Plot B2 (middle)

The following points can be made:

1. The soil water pressure at all depths is low indicating a near saturated soil (−10kPa is a typical pressure at field capacity) with only the soil at 150cm appearing to be consistently drier than field capacity.

2. For plots A1, B1 and B5 the 100cm readings are consistently more positive than those at 50cm depth. This may indicate a wetter layer at 100cm perhaps as a result of weathering or unloading effects or a lens of material of a different nature.

3. The drained (B) plots tend to have higher negative pressures at 150cm depth than do the undrained plots, indicating that the drains seem to be effective in reducing soil moisture at this depth.

4. There is a clear response in the tensiometer data to rainfall with a short lag time of around 24 hours for the 25cm depth (mainly a function of the sampling time). The response is less clear at greater depth and the time lag increases to 72 hours at 150cm.

5. Over the winter period the soils became progressively wetter at depth; by the end of January 1995 positive pore water pressures were recorded at some depths in all plots. The effect of the drains is maintained at 150cm, but not at other depths.

Figure 6.5 shows midday tensiometer readings for the middle instrument nest for plot B5 for the period 25 February 1995–27 April 1995. Again the trends shown are typical for all the plots. Key observations here relate to the values at 25cm. From the spring period beginning in April 1995, probably due to a dry spell enhancing the effects of increasing evapo-transpiration at the onset of the growing season, the soil is drying out rapidly at this depth. The drying continues throughout the summer extending to all depths except 150cm. At 150cm the soil remains at or near to field capacity.

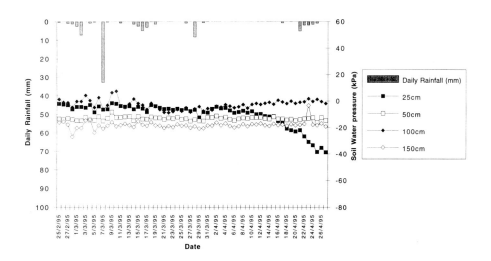

Figure 6.5 Midday tensiometer data for Plot B5 (middle)

The soil water pressure influences the effective stresses within the soil. It does not, however, provide information on water movement through the soil which is governed by the soil water potential which relates the pressure at various points to a fixed hydraulic reference datum such as the ground surface (see Glossary). Wherever the potential differs from point to point, the water experiences a force which tends to make it move from positions of greater to lower potential. By plotting the soil water potential against depth, a gradient of potential can be drawn which gives both the magnitude and direction of the water-moving force. The rate of water movement over the potential gradient is determined by the permeability of the soil, which depends on the proportion of conducting pores and degree of saturation. When a soil drains to field capacity, its permeability is often reduced to less than 1/100th of its permeability at saturation. In an unsaturated soil, the rate of water flow along a potential gradient is likely to be very slow, regardless of the magnitude of the differences in potential. The permeability of heavy clay soils like those of the Longham Wood Cutting is extremely low. This should be borne in mind when interpreting the significance of the soil water potential gradients identified from the tensiometer data.

Figure 6.6 shows soil water potential gradients for the storm of 27 October to 1 November 1994 for the top slope tensiometer nests in the undrained plot A2 and the drained plot B2. For plot A2 there is a clear response to rainfall in the top 25cm, with water draining down from above and by capillary rise from the saturated zone around 100cm. Below 100cm water is draining down through the soil profile. The change in gradient at 50cm suggests that at this level there is no water movement and a plane of zero flux exists. There is a similar layer at 100cm which marks the boundaries between water being attracted upwards to the 50cm level and water continuing to drain down the profile. Planes of zero flux are often indicators of an active root zone drawing water at this depth. Roots are unlikely to be the cause of the zero flux planes in this instance, however, as the vegetation has only just become established and few roots have penetrated to below 25cm depth.

Plot A2 (top) 27 October - 1 November 1994

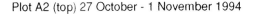

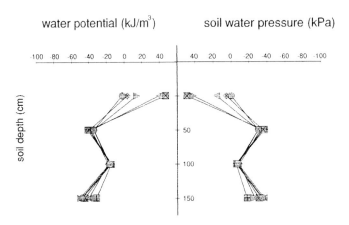

Plot B2 (top) 27 October - 1 November 1994

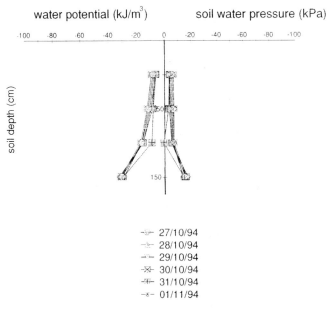

- 27/10/94
- 28/10/94
- 29/10/94
- 30/10/94
- 31/10/94
- 01/11/94

Figure 6.6 Tensiometer data for a winter storm

The gradient for plot B2 reveals that the soil is wetter than field capacity down to 150cm where the drains may be influencing the soil moisture. Water is moving up the profile from the plane of zero flux at 100cm, but the differences in potential are so small and the daily changes so slight that any movement is minimal. Below 100cm water drains down the profile towards the land drains. Both plots reveal a wetter layer at 100cm which may indicate the presence of a wetting front from a previous rainy period.

Figure 6.7 shows gradients for 1 – 6 July 1995 for the middle tensiometer nests on plots A2 and B2. Both clearly show the seasonal effects of a dry hot summer as the soils are drier than field capacity at all depths. For plot A2 the missing values at 25cm are probably a result of the surface soil becoming too dry for the tensiometers to function. There is a general trend in this plot for water to move up the profile from 150cm as a result of the high evapo-transpiration rates at the surface, though for 3, 4 and 6 July there is some evidence of downward drainage from 50cm to 100cm. Again the differences in water potential on these days are so slight that there will be only minimal water movement.

Plot A2 (middle) 1 - 6 July 1995

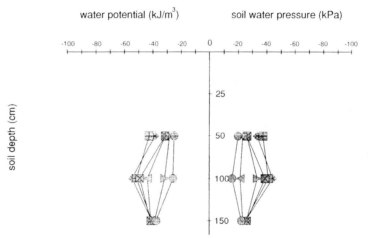

Plot B2 (middle) 1 - 6 July 1995

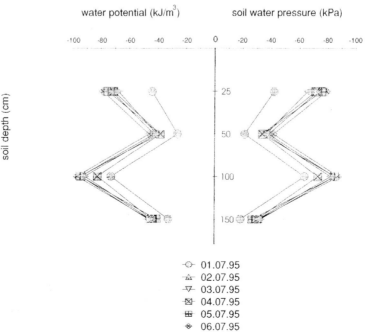

-○- 01.07.95
-△- 02.07.95
-▽- 03.07.95
-⊠- 04.07.95
-⊞- 05.07.95
-◈- 06.07.95

Figure 6.7 Tensiometer data for a drying period in summer

Plot B2 clearly has two distinct wetter layers, and 50cm and 150cm, with the layer at 150cm only just drier than field capacity. Water is moving up from 50cm and down to 100cm. The wetter layer at 50cm may again indicate the position of a previous wetting front moving through the profile.

By July 1995, roots had developed on both plots to 25cm depth with some extending to 45cm. These could be drawing water up the profile from 50cm on both plots. The usefulness of soil water potential analysis will become more apparent when the vegetation is fully established as the planes of zero flux could mark the extent of the active rooting zone, and, by assessing the angle of gradient, the efficiency of the roots at removing water from the soil may be estimated. More detailed analysis of the data should be able to identify how the different plots respond to rainfall events in terms of speed of drainage, and may identify layers within the plots where drainage is impeded.

Figure 6.8 shows an example of typical diurnal variation in tensiometer data for two plots over 24 hours on 28 October 1994. There is little change over the 24-hour period with only small variations in soil water pressure. This is normal and representative of areas with little vegetation. There is very little plant transpiration to influence the soil water status, and daily changes in evaporation do not result in changes in soil water pressure below the top 5cm. Also with soils such as these with low hydraulic conductivity even rainfall during a 24-hour period does not have a large immediate effect on soil water pressure.

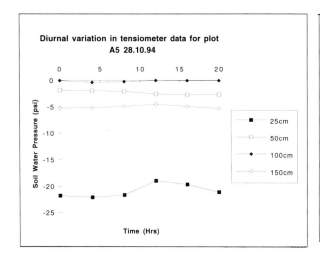
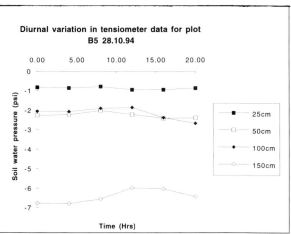

Figure 6.8 Diurnal variations in tensiometer data

Figure 6.9 shows contours of soil water potential at the four depths of measurement for 27 October 1994. By interpretation of such figures, it is possible to identify the spatial pattern of potential water movement over the slope in three dimensions, i.e. movement across and down the slope at a given depth and through the soil profile from one depth to another. The spacing of the contours represents the potential energy of flow with water moving from areas of high to low soil water potential.

On 27 October 1994, the water potential values for each depth reflect those shown in Figure 6.6 with potential being high at 25cm, decreasing at 50cm, increasing slightly at

100cm and decreasing again at 150cm. Considerable variability exists across the slope at the 25cm depth on the A5 and A2 plots. High water potential occurs at the top of A5 and on the lower slope of A2; strongly negative values exist in the middle of A5. Thus a potential gradient exists for water movement from the top of plots A5 and A2 towards the centre of A5. In contrast, the water potential values for the A1 and all the B plots are reasonably uniform and there is little potential for water movement.

At the 50cm depth, water potential is lowest at the bottom of A1 and at the top of A1 and A2. The range in potential values over all six plots is much lower than that at the 25cm depth. Considering the contours at the 25cm and 50cm depths together, the potential exists for water in the soil at the 25cm depth at the top of A1 and the middle of B1 to drain down to the 50cm layer. The potential for water movement to the 100cm depth is limited because of the slightly higher potential values at that depth compared with those at 50cm; as stated earlier, there may be a remnant of a previous wetting front at 100cm. There is potential for some downward water movement, however, to the bottom of plot B1. Further downward movement would be expected towards the bottom of B2 and B5 at the 150cm depth.

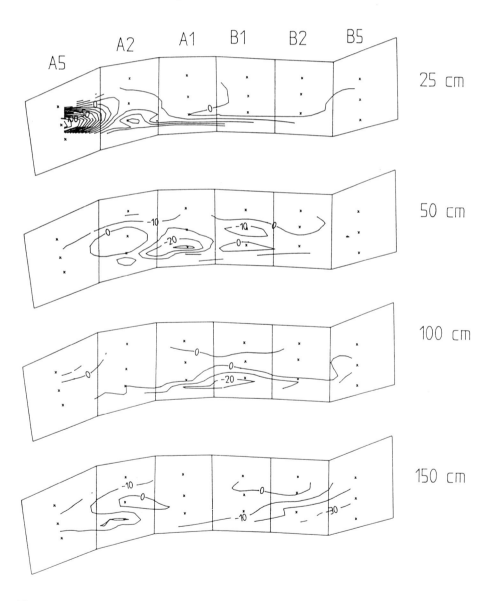

Figure 6.9 Spatial distribution of soil water potential across primary plots at different depths

The contour plots thus indicate the potential for water movement, not only downslope or vertically downwards through the soil profile, but also across the slope. On the 27 October 1994 there was potential for water movement diagonally from the top of plot A1 at 25cm to the bottom of plot B1 at 100cm and the bottom of B2 and B5 at 150cm as the wetting front moved through the soil. Similar contour plots over a sequence of days would determine whether that movement occurred. If successions of contour plots showed such directional flow to be repeated regularly, they would indicate potential areas of water concentration and, depending on the pore water pressures obtained, would indicate locations of higher risk of slope instability. Changes in the contour plots with the growth of vegetation would indicate whether bio-engineering was effective in reducing the risk in such locations.

6.2.2 Neutron probe data

The soil moisture content profile was determined with the neutron probe on the following dates:

19 October 1994, 1 December 1994, 20 January 1995, 24 February 1995, 26 April 1995, 23 May 1995, 29 June 1995 and 10 August 1995.

The probe reading was calibrated to give the volumetric moisture content. This was converted to gravimetric moisture content as follows:

$$\text{Gravimetric Moisture Content} = \frac{\text{Volumetric Moisture Content}}{\text{Dry Density}}$$

An average dry density of $1.48Mg/m^3$ was used in the conversion.

Figure 6.10 shows the neutron probe data for 19 October 1994 converted to a gravimetric moisture content for plots A1, A2, A5, B1, B2 and B5.

The neutron probe-derived moisture contents reveal no clear differences between the treatments or position on the slope and show a slight increase in moisture content with depth. This is not contradictory to the tensiometer data as a neutron probe measures absolute water content whereas a tensiometer measures soil water pressure. These are two entirely different soil properties and not directly comparable.

Figure 6.11 shows the Neutron probe data for 24 February 1995 and clearly indicates that the soil is wetter than in the October of the previous year. Again there is no clear difference between plots, though in general the sites at the bottom of the slope seem to be slightly wetter than those in the middle and top of the slope.

Figure 6.12 shows the Neutron probe data for 10 August 1995 and there are visible differences between plots A5 and A2 and the other plots which appear to be wetter below 80cm. There is no apparent difference between position on the slope, but for all treatments the soils clearly become wetter with depth.

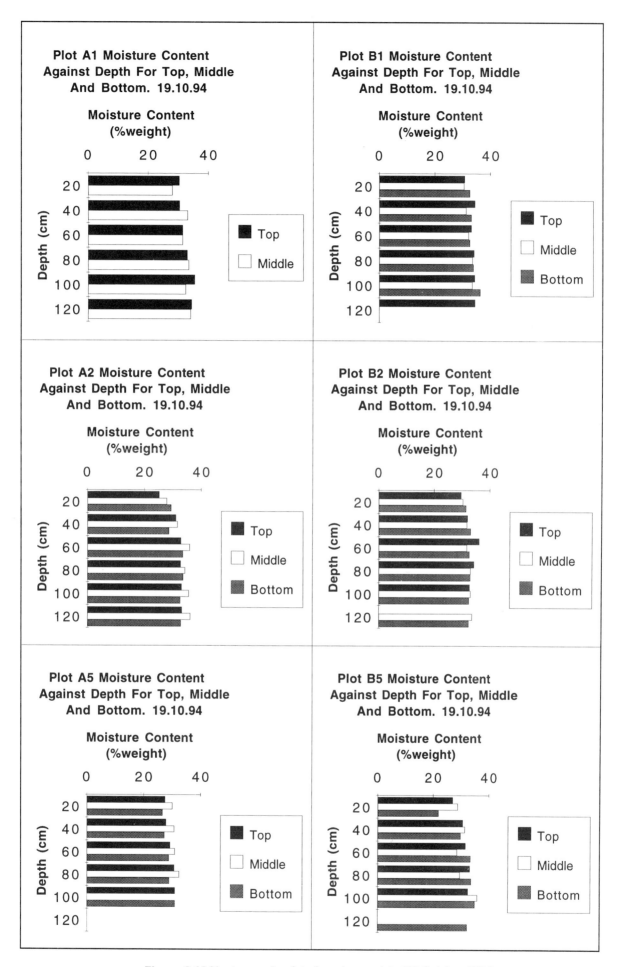

Figure 6.10 Neutron probe data for primary plots (19 October 1994)

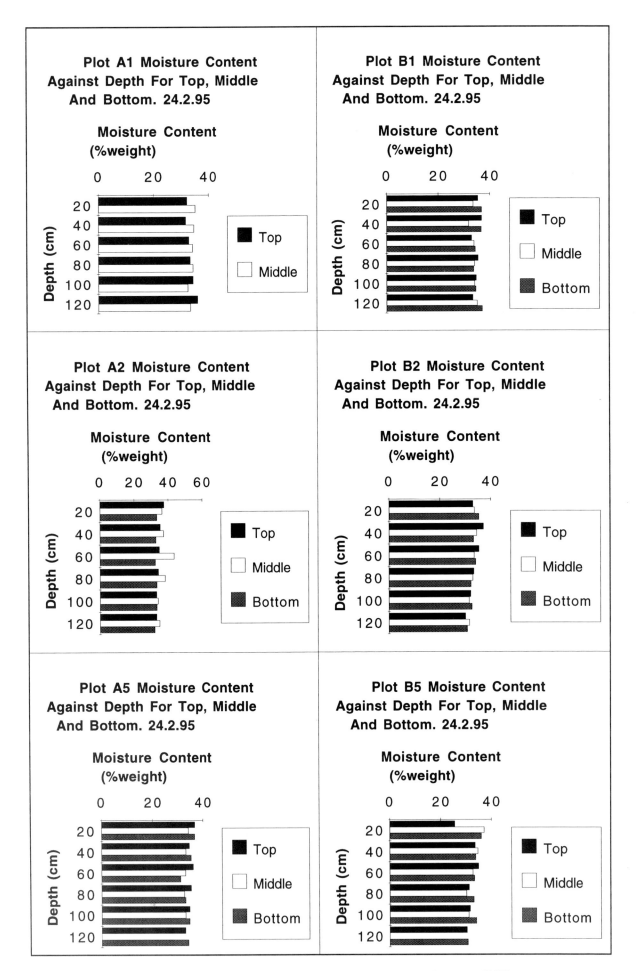

Figure 6.11 Neutron probe data for primary plots (24 February 1995)

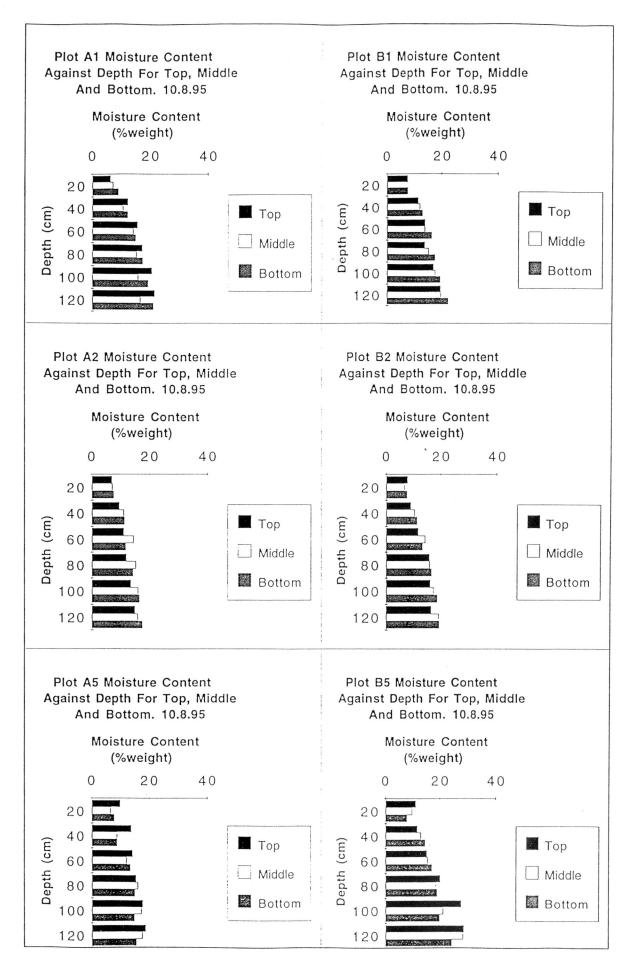

Figure 6.12 Neutron probe data for primary plots (10 August 1995)

6.3 GEOTECHNICAL RESULTS

6.3.1 General

The results of the geotechnical testing are presented in summary form on Figures 6.13 and 6.14. Complete results including tests taken during the investigation and construction of the Longham Wood Cutting are available in the Data Appendix.

Data plotted illustrates the changes in moisture content, shear strength by penetrometer (shear strength = scale reading/2), shear strength by hand vane (uncorrected scale reading), and Mackintosh Probe results (blows/100 mm) for three test locations in each of two primary plots (A5 and B5).

The results of the testing are discussed in the following sections.

6.3.2 Standpipes

The standpipe readings, plotted in Figure 6.15 were consistent throughout the monitoring period and demonstrated a water table fluctuating seasonally between ground level and approximately 2m depth.

The results are not directly comparable with the tensiometers, as the standpipes average water pressure over the depths of the filter installation. They require considerable volume of water to operate and may be susceptible to inflow of surface water due to problems with the clay seal shrinking away from the pipe.

The standpipe readings did not indicate differences in water level between drained plots (standpipes P3 and P4) and the undrained plots (standpipes P1 and P2).

6.3.3 Slip plane indicators

The plumb rod could be inserted into all access tubes indicating that no significant ground movement occurred over the monitoring period.

6.3.4 Mackintosh probes

The Mackintosh Probe proved a relatively quick and easy test to carry out with minimal disturbance to the site. The blow count (per 100mm) clearly reflected the changing state of the soil on a seasonal basis down to approximately 1m in depth. There is no formal correlation between the Mackintosh Probe blow count and other soil parameters but it is possible to derive an empirical relationship from the data now available. For example:

$$\text{Vane shear strength (kN/m}^2) = 4 \times \text{probe blow count (blows/100mm)}$$

Further results are necessary before this relationship may be used with any certainty.

6.3.5 Core sampling

The use of the geodrive window sampler proved reasonably successful in obtaining core samples for root count, hand vane and penetrometer readings on site and for taking samples for laboratory determination of the moisture content. It was not found practical to use a plastic liner within the sampler and depth of sampling was sometimes restricted to approximately 1.3m in the harder soils. Testing depths had to be adjusted slightly to suit the position of the window.

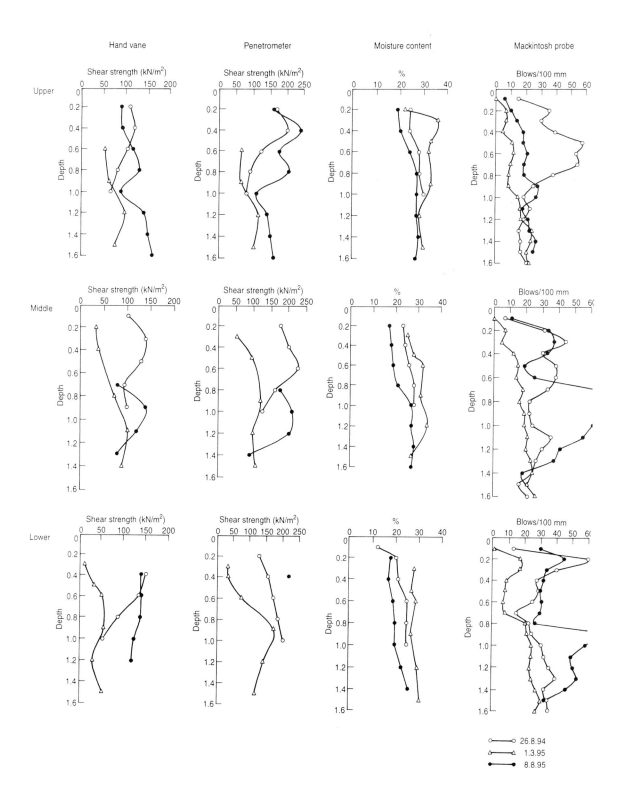

Figure 6.13 Geotechnical data for plot A5

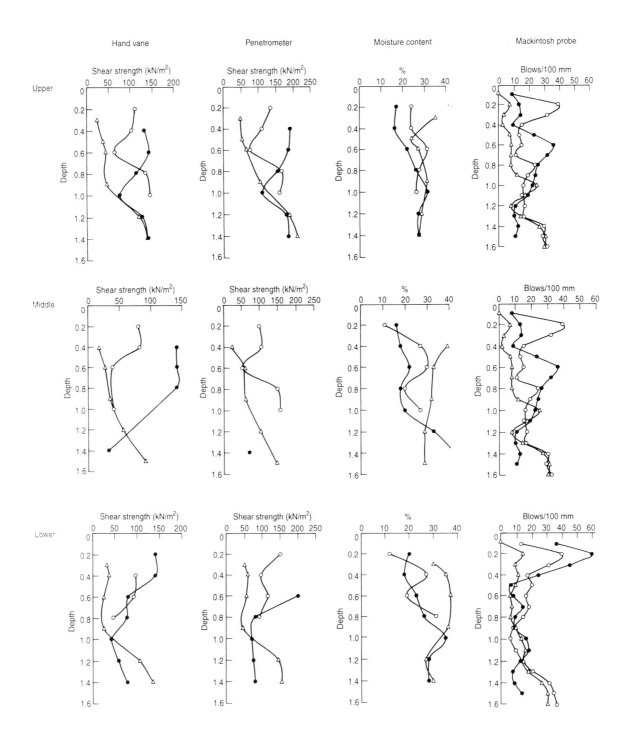

Figure 6.14 Geotechnical data for plot B5

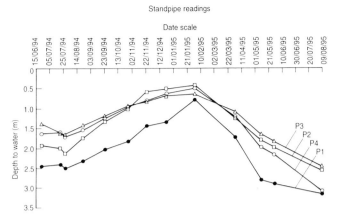

Standpipe readings

Figure 6.15 Plot of piezometer readings (refer to Figure 5.1 for piezometer locations)

The main concerns with the geodrive sampling were the destructive effects on the vegetation and soil regime. It was inevitable that the 2-person geodrive teams and specialist supervisors together with the rods and equipment required would cause trampling and temporary damage to the vegetation at the test locations, particularly during wet conditions.

It is intended to reduce the amount of core sampling for future phases of the monitoring to that necessary for root observation only to a maximum depth of 1m. This should enable lighter equipment to be used with reduced site damage.

6.3.6 Vane and penetrometer strength and moisture content

The shear strength measured by hand vane and penetrometer was considered to be sufficiently accurate for the study purposes recognising that there will always be an inherent variability within the natural Gault clay. In general the moisture content and strength data show consistent results which also relate to the Mackintosh Probe data as described in Section 6.3.4.

There was no significant difference in the shear strengths and moisture contents measured for the drained (B plots) and undrained (A plots) sections of the site.

6.3.7 Correlation between the neutron probe data and oven dried moisture content determinations

A correlation between the neutron probe moisture content and the field-measured gravimetric moisture content is difficult to make because the soil samples for the latter determinations were not taken on the same dates as the neutron probe data. It is also physically impossible to sample the same area using two different methods, so samples for gravimetric moisture determination were taken as close to the access tubes as possible without destroying the plots. This will introduce an aspect of spatial variability into any correlation. Nevertheless, a correlation was attempted for the two closest sample dates which were 7 – 8 August 1995 for the gravimetric moisture contents, and 10 August 1995 for the neutron probe data. The results in Figure 6.16 shows a reasonable 1-to-1 relationship between the two sets of data. The samples collected for gravimetric moisture content determination were slightly wetter than those determined by the neutron probe. A more detailed comparison at different locations within plot B5 is presented in Figure 6.17. This shows the changes in the moisture content between summer and winter seasons and the variation at each stage between the upper, middle and lower monitoring locations within the plot. The relationship between neutron probe and oven-dried moisture contents is close enough to recommend that only neutron probe determination is carried out in future.

Figure 11. Neutron Probe Moisture Content Against Oven
Moisture Content

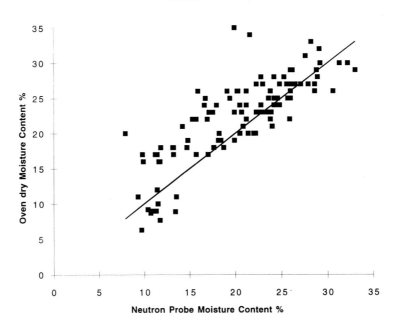

Figure 6.16 Neutron probe moisture content vs. oven-derived moisture content

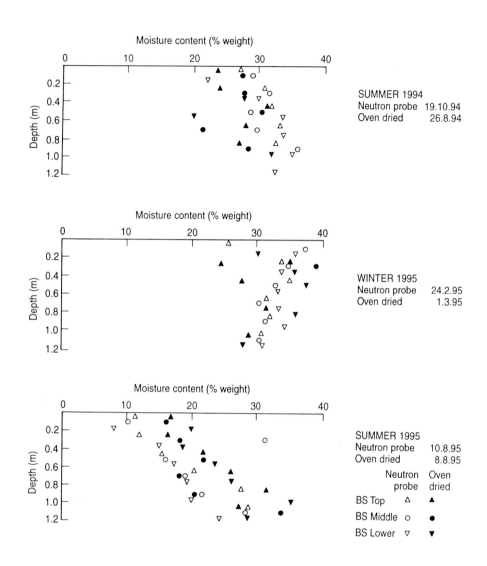

Figure 6.17 Detailed comparison of neutron probe and oven-dried moisture contents for different seasons and at different testing locations within plot B5

7   Stability analysis

7.1   THEORETICAL ANALYSIS

There are a number of methods for assessing the stability of soil slopes, all of which involve certain simplifying assumptions to obtain a calculated factor of safety. The most commonly used approach is the limit equilibrium technique with the factor of safety, F, simply defined for a particular slip surface as:

$$F = \frac{\text{shear resistance along a slip surface}}{\text{shear force acting along the slip surface}}$$

The 'method of slices' is well established and various methods which may be used to demonstrate the effects of vegetation are described by Coppin and Richards (1990). The simple method of Greenwood (1983), given in Coppin and Richards (1990), is readily adapted for analysing the effects of vegetation on any slip surface, whether circular or non-circular.

The main influences of vegetation on a slope are summarised in Figure 7.1 taken from Coppin and Richards (1990). The terms used in the stability analysis are defined in Figure 7.1.

The factor of safety of the cutting slope at Longham Wood has been considered for a series of potential slab slides at depths of 0.3m (base of topsoil), 0.5m, 1.0m and 1.5m below ground level. These correspond with the depths of the installed tensiometers. This simplified analysis is illustrated in Figure 7.2.

Circular and composite slip surfaces may also be analysed if relevant as field results are obtained. The soil strength parameters may be considered in terms of effective stress parameters (c', Ø') or total stress parameters (Cu, Ø = 0) as appropriate.

The calculated factors of safety for the slab slides, which were determined without considering vegetation effects, are given in Table 7.1. These are based on the assumptions noted.

Table 7.1 Calculated factors of safety for 1:3 slope at Longham Wood without considering effects of vegetation

Depth (m below ground level)	F (where c' = 1.5, Ø' = 17 and r_u = 0)	F (where c' = 1.5, Ø' = 17 and r_u = 0.5)	F (where Cu = 20 and Ø = 0)
0.3	1.75	1.29	-
0.5	1.42	0.96	6.68
1.0	1.17	0.71	3.34
1.5	1.09	0.63	2.23

Note:
$$r_u = \frac{u}{\gamma h_z}, \text{ where } \gamma = \text{soil bulk density}$$

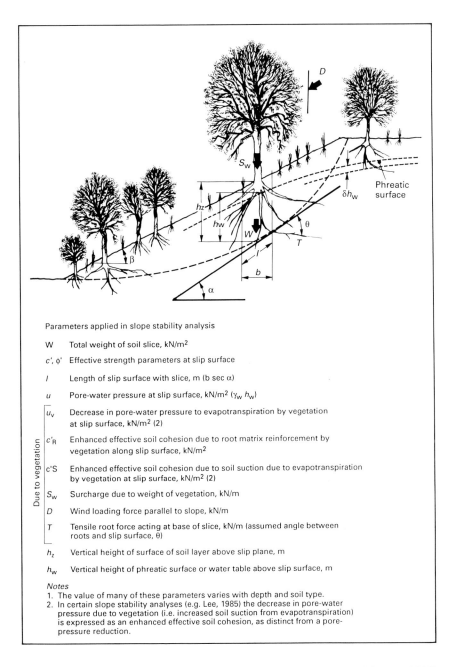

Parameters applied in slope stability analysis

W   Total weight of soil slice, kN/m²

c', ϕ' Effective strength parameters at slip surface

l Length of slip surface with slice, m (b sec α)

u Pore-water pressure at slip surface, kN/m² (γ_w h_w)

u_v Decrease in pore-water pressure to evapotranspiration by vegetation
         at slip surface, kN/m² (2)

c'_R Enhanced effective soil cohesion due to root matrix reinforcement by
         vegetation along slip surface, kN/m²

$c'S$ Enhanced effective soil cohesion due to soil suction due to evapotranspiration
         by vegetation at slip surface, kN/m² (2)

S_w Surcharge due to weight of vegetation, kN/m

D Wind loading force parallel to slope, kN/m

T Tensile root force acting at base of slice, kN/m (assumed angle between
         roots and slip surface, θ)

h_z Vertical height of surface of soil layer above slip plane, m

h_w Vertical height of phreatic surface or water table above slip surface, m

Notes
1. The value of many of these parameters varies with depth and soil type.
2. In certain slope stability analyses (e.g. Lee, 1985) the decrease in pore-water
   pressure due to vegetation (i.e. increased soil suction from evapotranspiration)
   is expressed as an enhanced effective soil cohesion, as distinct from a pore-
   pressure reduction.

Figure 7.1 The influences of vegetation on a slope (Coppin and Richards, 1990)

In reality, as described by Greenwood *et.al* (1985), the parameters c', Ø' and r_u are likely to change with depth due to restraints of penetration of weathering and localised water table effects.

The basic stability equation (Greenwood 1983) is:

$$F = \frac{\sum \left[c'b\sec\alpha + (W - ub)\cos\alpha \tan\phi' \right]}{\sum W \sin\alpha}$$

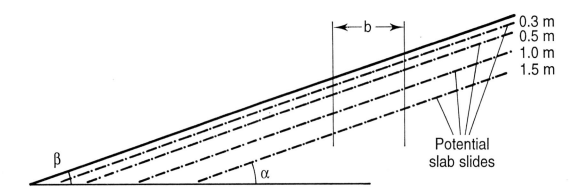

Figure 7.2 Simplified analysis of Longham Wood Cutting (after Greenwood, *et al*, 1985)

This equation is easily modified to include vegetation factors (Richards and Coppin 1990):

$$F = \frac{\sum \left\{ (c'+c'_R)b\sec\alpha + \left[((w + S_w) - (u - u_V)b)\cos\alpha - D\sin(\alpha - \beta) + T\sin\theta \right]\tan\phi' + T\cos\theta \right.}{\sum \left[(W + S_w)\sin\alpha + D\cos(\alpha - \beta) \right]}$$

and is further simplified by the assumption in Figure 7.2 that the angles α and β are equal, such that the terms $\sin(\alpha-\beta)$ and $\cos(\alpha-\beta)$ become 0 and 1 respectively.

7.2 THEORETICAL EFFECTS OF VEGETATION

It is anticipated that the vegetation planted at Longham Wood Cutting should eventually be effective in the following ways relating to the parameters given in Figure 7.1.

u_V Willows in particular, with high leaf areas, rapid growth and high water demand will reduce water pressures. Assume that u_V may attain a value of 3.0kN/m².

c'_r Tap rooted forbs within the grass/forb treatment and the deep rooting potential of the tree and shrub species will increase soil cohesion. Assume that c'_r has a value of 2.0kN/m² and therefore c' increases from 1.5 to 3.5kN/m².

Sw The weight of the vegetation will be minimal in relation to soil weights and can therefore be disregarded.

D   The only vegetation that may have a wind loading effect would be the willows. However these are to be subject to a coppice management regime so wind load factors will not be significant.

T   The deep roots, such as the tap roots from shrubs such as the gorse, should eventually develop a tensile root force of up to 5kN/m. Assume these act at an average of $45°$ to the slip plane, i.e. $\theta = 45°$.

The vegetation could, in theory, have a significant effect on the factor of safety. This is illustrated for the slip surface at 1m depth in Table 7.2.

Table 7.2 Example of calculated factors of safety at 1m depth due to possible effects of vegetation

Condition	Parameters				Factor of safety
no vegetation (taken from Table 7.1)	$c' = 1.5$	$\phi' = 17$	$r_u = 0.5$		0.71
vegetation effect					
a) reduced water pressure	$c' = 1.5$	$\phi' = 17$	$\mathbf{r_u = 0.4}$		0.80
b) tap rooted forbs	$\mathbf{c' = 3.5}$	$\phi' = 17$	$r_u = 0.5$		1.04
c) deep roots	$c' = 1.5$	$\phi' = 17$	$r_u = 0.5$	$\mathbf{T = 5\ kN/m}$	0.86
Combined effect (a+b+c)	$\mathbf{c' = 3.5}$	$\phi' = 17$	$\mathbf{r_u = 0.4}$	$\mathbf{T = 5\ kN/m}$	1.28

Note: Applied effect of vegetation shown with parameters in bold type.

7.3 ACTUAL EFFECTS OF VEGETATION

The Gault clay in the slope at Longham Wood Cutting exhibits reasonable consistency as a material but inevitably with a natural material geotechnical properties vary from location to location.

The geotechnical data taken over the monitoring period has highlighted seasonal variations in the moisture and groundwater regime within the Gault clay slope. These natural and seasonal conditions are at present masking any effects due to the vegetation. As the vegetation continues to become established it is expected that a modification to the seasonal changes will be detected by the instrumentation and monitoring regime.

8 Summary and recommendations

8.1 SUMMARY

A cutting in Gault clay located on the M20 motorway in Kent and with a history of shallow seated slope failures has been selected as a suitable site to demonstrate the potential value of vegetation to improve slope stability.

The primary site was steepened to 1 in 3 and divided into 6 plots. Three different types of vegetation – willows and alders, gorse and broom mix, and forbs and grasses – were planted in 3 undrained plots. The same vegetation types were planted in 3 further plots with 3m deep counterfort drains installed. Other vegetation types were planted in varying topsoil thicknesses in a series of secondary demonstration plots on the 1 in 6 cutting slope.

Geotechnical and hydrological instrumentation was installed and a monitoring and testing programme established.

In the 2-year period 1994–5 the vegetation has become established with little loss during particularly dry summers.

The monitoring programme has been successful in demonstrating the seasonal changes in the soil parameters. It is too soon after planting to identify parameter changes due to the effects of the vegetation, although the monitoring regime undertaken demonstrates that it would be possible to identify such effects.

8.2 RECOMMENDATIONS

Monitoring of the vegetation and its effects on the geotechnical parameters should be continued. It would be expected that the significant effects of root reinforcement of the soil mass and control of soil moisture by the vegetation will start to become apparent 3 to 5 years after planting and monitoring over a 10-year period is recommended. This would be consistent with the observed characteristics of clay slopes, of the kind used, to suffer geotechnical failures after 5–10 years. This first stage of the study has provided valuable experience in specification, monitoring and maintenance of a range of vegetation types.

Hydrological testing by tensiometers and neutron probes should be continued on a similar frequency to that carried out to date.

The physical geotechnical sampling and testing is particularly destructive and tends to damage vegetation in the vicinity of the monitoring point. Correlation between the moisture content determined by oven drying of samples and by the less destructive neutron probe method is generally good. Other soil properties may be derived from the moisture content. It is therefore proposed to reduce the physical core sampling to that necessary for root count purposes only and to rely on the neutron probe results supplemented by Mackintosh Probing to assess the geotechnical conditions.

Consideration should be given to alternative ways of monitoring the effects of the vegetation on the soil with minimal physical disturbance.

It may be appropriate after approximately 5 years to excavate a series of trial trenches to provide detailed records of root growth and direct measurement of the soil parameters on blocks affected by the roots. Considerable disturbance and vegetation damage in the vicinity of the trenches would have to be accepted in order to obtain the precise data.

The reliability of plant growth and root development over the years and seasonal die-back are factors which require further definition so that engineers may have reasonable confidence in the enhanced soil parameters used in the stability analysis.

In addition to the further monitoring recommended at the existing site, it is also recommended that some qualitative data be obtained from established sites in other locations to gauge the long-term effects of the vegetation.

References

BARKER, D.H. (1986)
Biodegradable geotextiles for erosion control and slope stabilisation. *Civil Engineering*,
June 1986, 13–15.

COPPIN, N. J. and RICHARDS, I. G. (1990)
Use of Vegetation in Civil Engineering, CIRIA publication, Butterworths.

FARRAR, D. M. (1984)
*Long-term Changes in Pore Water Pressure within an Embankment Built of London
Clay,*
Transport and Road Research Laboratory Report.

GRAY, D. H. (1978)
Role of Woody Vegetation in reinforcing soils and stability slopes.
In: *Symp. Soil Reinforcing and Stabilising Techniques.* New South Wales Institute of
Technology, pp. 253–306.

GREENWOOD, J.R. (1983)
A simple approach to slope stability, Ground Engineering, 16(4), 45-98

GREENWOOD, J. R., HOLT, P. A. and HERRICK G. W. (1985)
Shallow Slips in Highway Embankments Constructed of Over-consolidated Clay. Proc.
symp. Failures in Earthworks, Paper 6, 79–92, ICE London.

JOHNSON, P.E. (1985)
*Maintenance and Repair of Highway Embankments: Studies of Seven Methods of
Treatment,* Transport and Road Research Laboratory, Research Report 30.

LEE, I.W.Y. (1985)
A review of vegetative slope stabilisation, *Journal Hong Kong Institute of Engineering*,
3(7), 9–21.

NORWEST HOLST SOIL ENGINEERING LTD (1989)
Site Investigation Report, M20 Improvement Junctions 5–8.

PARSONS, A. W. and PERRY, J. (1985)
Slope stability problems in ageing highway earthworks,
Proc. Symp. Failures in Earthworks
ICE (London).

PERRY, J. (1989)
A Survey of Slope Condition on Motorway Earthworks in England and Wales, Transport
and Road Research Laboratory Report RR199.

RICHARDS, MOOREHEAD and LAING, TRAVERS MORGAN and SILSOE
COLLEGE (1992)
Field Evaluation and Demonstration Sites for Bio-engineering and Bank Protection.

Appendix A1 Literature review

SUMMARY

This outline review identifies the particular problem of shallow-seated slip failures in clay embankments and cuttings, and describes the failure mechanisms as currently understood. It summarises the conventional repair techniques and preventative measures available. The potential for the use of vegetation to strengthen such slopes is discussed, and examples of techniques used elsewhere are reported. Further sections identify the vegetation characteristics required and possible suitable species, and methods used to measure and monitor key parameters of ground conditions. Finally, a summary of other related experimental work is presented which identifies the lack of experimental experience in the application of bio-engineering to shallow-seated slope failures.

A1.1   INTRODUCTION

A1.1.1   Background

The book 'Use of Vegetation in Civil Engineering' was published in 1990 as the outcome of a CIRIA research project aimed at providing technical guidance to practising engineers on the use of vegetation as an engineering material. To encourage the uptake of these promising new techniques, CIRIA initiated an evaluation programme relating primarily to the use of vegetation in slope stabilisation, by establishing trial/demonstration sites in suitable locations.

The project 'Field evaluation and demonstration sites for bio-engineering and bank protection' commenced with a limited literature review and outline design of the demonstration sites. The literature review is reported in this document.

A1.1.2   Subject area

CIRIA has identified the stabilisation of earth slopes against shallow failure (associated with urban and infrastructure development) as a key market area for the use of vegetation in civil engineering, together with the control of surface erosion of earth surfaces (associated with various types of development).

Vegetative control of erosion, and specialised techniques for the establishment of vegetation on easily eroded sites, have been widely adopted by the industry as a result, in part, of the commercial availability of materials such as seeded and unseeded erosion control mats, geotextiles and the like.

The current demonstration project therefore concentrates on techniques for stabilisation against shallow failure, where the use of vegetation has not yet been widely adopted and the relevant techniques are less developed or well known.

A1.2   SLOPE FAILURES IN CLAY EMBANKMENTS AND CUTTINGS

A1.2.1   The nature of the problem

Shallow-seated slope failures are defined for the purpose of this project, as mass soil movements with a slip surface no more than 2m below the surface of the ground. The soil movement may be translational, rotational, or more commonly a combination of the two.

Deeper-seated failures are excluded from this project since they are not considered to be susceptible to stabilisation by vegetation.

A1.2.2   The extent of the problem

Shallow-seated slope failures have occurred in many locations in Britain where naturally occurring over-consolidated clays have been exposed in cuttings or re-used in embankments. Particular problems have been experienced along major road routes where the need to minimise land-take has led to the adoption of steep side slopes. Parsons and Perry (1985), reported a survey of motorway slopes in which failures were recorded as a percentage of the total length of slope constructed of each soil material. Over a total surveyed length of 300km of motorway in various geologies, almost 15km of cutting and embankment slope had failed. Slopes, both cutting and embankment, constructed in Gault Clay geology had significantly higher failure rates (9.7% and 9.1%) than any other geology surveyed.

The A45 and M11 north of Cambridge suffered over 30 embankment failures since their construction in the late 1970s (Johnson, 1985). These failures were typically shallow translational slides in the over-consolidated Gault Clay used to construct embankments. Typical repair costs have been £10–15,000 (1980s prices) per failure for the excavation and granular replacement method (Greenwood, Holt and Herrick, 1985). Clearly, the national cost of repairing such failures is considerable, and an understanding of the causes and possible means of prevention is highly desirable.

A1.2.3   The mechanism of failure

The failure problem described in Section A1.2 is particularly common in over-consolidated clays, that is, 'clays which have gained strength by consolidation under a heavy excess overburden pressure or by dessication due to evaporation or the growth of vegetation' (BS6031: 1981).

Excavation for a cutting wholly or partly relieves stress on the remaining soil, leading to a reduction in pore water pressure within the slope and a temporary increase in strength and stability. Recharge of water from rainfall or groundwater gradually increases pore water pressures to equilibrium, reducing soil strength and slope stability. (BS6031: 1981). The construction of an embankment in similar materials causes a temporary increase in pore water pressures due to increased stress. It is accepted practice to limit the rate of embankment building to allow pore water pressures to dissipate. Greenwood et al (1985) state that the convention of designing embankments using data for undrained soils, and assuming a progressive increase in soil strength with time, is not necessarily applicable for some over-consolidated clays.

Detailed geotechnical explanations of the physical processes involved in cutting and embankment construction and deep failure are given in various publications (e.g. BS6031: 1981, DOE 1991). Greenwood et al (1985) proposed the following mechanism to explain the occurrence of shallow failures (typically 1.0 to 1.5m depth) in embankment within a few years of construction. Their proposal drew on observations recorded by others including Parsons and Perry (1985), Farrar (1978, 1984) and Anderson and Kneale (1980). Greenwood et al note that over-consolidated clay is excavated and placed in embankments, with clay from deeper horizons tending to form the surface layers of embankments. This clay has the greatest suction as the greatest stress relief has taken place. Water from rainfall, road drainage, sub-base drainage, tension or shrinkage cracks and tree planting pits steadily or seasonally reduces this suction, increasing pore water pressure and reducing strength until failure occurs. As this re-wetting progresses from the surface downwards the failure is almost always at shallow depth (1–1.5m depth).

This mechanism is consistent with measurements by Farrar (1984) showing positive pore water pressures at shallow depths, and with observations by, among others Garrett and Wale (1985) that failures are frequently associated with periods of prolonged heavy rainfall. In 1991, Crabb and Atkinson reported their detailed study of the soil mechanics of such failures. They concluded that failures of cut and fill slopes in such clays occurred typically by slipping along planes parallel to the surface, at depths of 1 to 2m where pore water pressures were typically close to zero. The critical (or fully softened) strength was found to be a good guide to the assessment of slope stability. Greenwood *et al* (1985) presented factor of safety calculations showing that failures at greater depths (i.e. greater than about 1.5m) were unlikely since a) greater overburden depth restricts softening, b) poor permeability restricts deeper wetting, c) horizontal stress at depth contributes more reliably to shear resistance.

Parsons and Perry (1985) observed that failure rates were higher in less- steep cuttings and embankments of certain materials (including Gault Clay) than in the steepest slopes. They concluded that the steepest slopes are better able to shed surface water and so will take longer to reach the softened condition causing failure. Shallower slopes above a maximum 'safe' angle will absorb surface water more quickly and hence fail at a younger age.

A1.2.4   Design for 'safe' slopes

Parsons and Perry (1985) used data from their survey to calculate slope angles for each geology and slope height which would be expected to produce no more than 1% failure over the first 20 years. While these values were not intended to be used alone as a design guide, they suggest that much shallower slopes than those typically used in modern road construction might be appropriate if long-term stability is to be assured. Considerations of cost, land- take and environmental factors are likely to prevent the widespread use of such slopes (as shallow as lv:4h for Gault Clay), and so other slope stabilisation techniques will be required in many cases.

As a result of many repeated failures in cuttings along the M20 Maidstone bypass, particularly at Longham Wood Cutting, a detailed analysis was carried out by Kent County Council (Garret and Wale, 1985). From this it was initially proposed to re-grade the slope from 1 in 3 to 1 in 6 but this was abandoned on the grounds of land take and loss of tree screening. Subsequent proposals, to excavate the unstable clay and replace it with granular material within the original land- take, were carried out, illustrating the need for alternatives to shallow gradient design in many instances.

A1.3   CIVIL ENGINEERING METHODS OF SLOPE REPAIR AND STRENGTHENING

A1.3.1   Granular replacement

This method is currently the most widely used technique (Johnson 1985). The softened clay is removed and free-draining fill such as cobbles, beach shingle, as-raised gravel or broken brick is used to reinstate the profile. This permeable layer permits free water to drain from the clay surface preventing wetting and softening of the clay beneath. Unless a covering of topsoil is introduced and grassed- over, the technique can give rise to unsightly features. The method is relatively expensive at about £25/m3 of filled volume or typically £10–15,000 per repair (Greenwood et al, 1985).

A1.3.2   Alternative methods

Johnson (1985) and Greenwood et al (1985) reported a trial of alternative construction methods suitable for embankment or cutting construction or repair. These were:

a)   lime addition to replaced clay, to increase its strength

b)   geogrid reinforcement to create partly restrained envelopes of soil

c)   gabion wall, to produce a retained, shallower slope

d)   tyre wall, to produce a retained, shallower slope

e)   ground anchors with geogrid layer, to increase stress and stability

f)   rock ribs, acting as deep stone drains to reduce pore water pressure and increase strength.

Costs in the trial, carried out on the A45 near Cambridge, were compared with the 'control' treatment of granular replacement. Gabion walling proved substantially more expensive, geogrid reinforcement was the cheapest reinstatement method, and the rock rib preventative construction proved least expensive of all the methods trialled.

Garrett and Wale (1985) reported a similar trial at Horish Wood on the M20 in Gault Clay. Lime stabilisation, excavation/recompaction and deep counterfort drains cost respectively 0.5, 0.33 and 0.17 times the cost of granular replacement.

Barker (1991) described a geogrid reinforcement technique which used a flexible geogrid inserted in narrow vertical trenches, cut into existing cuttings or embankments in need of strengthening. The technique was considered appropriate where horizontal geotextile inclusions would be impractical.

A1.3.3   Surface stabilisation techniques

Many erosion-control systems have been developed, using combinations of vegetation and geotextiles. These products and their use were reviewed by Coppin and Richards (1990) and by Barker (1986). The use of surface-laid or shallow-buried geotextiles cannot directly contribute to the stabilisation of slopes which are prone to the failures described earlier in this review, but by assisting vegetation establishment where erosion is a problem, they have a valuable function in some situations. Cellular geotextiles are used particularly to restrain thick layers of soil placed on steep regraded slopes. Anchorage is provided by pinning into the underlying slope or burying the top of the geotextile. Although these products may restrain soil to a depth of 300mm or more they too offer no strengthening at the 1.0 to 1.5m depth typical of shallow failures in over-consolidated clays. Richards, Moorehead and Laing (1985) reviewed the use of vegetation and combined vegetative/structural slope protection systems for the shallow stabilisation of slopes, but this review dealt primarily with cuttings in rock and scree slopes. It specifically excluded slope failure problems.

A1.4   THE PROPERTIES AND FUNCTION OF VEGETATION

A1.4.1   Introduction

General reviews of plant growth requirements, the effects of established vegetation, and the functions of vegetation in bio- engineering have been prepared by various authors including Coppin and Richards (1990), Bache and MacAskill (1984), Gray (1978) and Schiechtl (1980). From these reviews it can be seen that vegetation could aid the stabilisation of shallow failure planes in clay slopes by performing the following functions:

- Removal of soil water by transpiration, reducing pore water pressures and counteracting the reduction of strength that wetting causes.

- Increasing shear strength by producing root fibres extended across the plane of potential shear failure.

- Buttressing, and soil arching between buttressed soil columns, due to trees and root columns acting as piles.

- Shading the surface to reduce shrinkage cracking which allows deep penetration of rainwater.

Each of these functions is discussed below.

A1.4.2   Removal of soil water

Vegetation can affect the stability of slopes by modifying the hydrological regime in the soil. Vegetation transpires soil water, and intercepts some rainfall for direct re-evaporation, thus maintaining drier soils and delaying the onset of saturated conditions in the soil (Gray 1978).

The ability of trees to deplete soil moisture to considerable depths is well known, and the consequences of this action in shrinkable clays near buildings have been studied in detail (Cutler and Richardson, 1989; Biddle, 1985). Biddle measured soil moisture in clay soils at varying distances from established trees to monitor seasonal changes within and beyond the root zone. Poplar was shown to be most efficient at removing water from a large soil volume. In October, the London clay soil beneath the canopy of the tree (0.8 x tree height) ranged from 42% moisture by volume at 3.5m depth to 33% moisture at 0.5m depth. Soil beyond the canopy (1.8 x tree height) had moisture contents of 47% and 45% at these depths. In late April, soil within the canopy still had a moisture content of 42% below 1.5m depth, but a moisture content of 44–46% above that depth. Beyond the canopy, the April soil moisture matched the October values.

From this data it can be seen that during the summer a mature Poplar significantly depletes the soil moisture to a considerable depth. It creates a column of permanently drier soil, and reduces the depth to which winter re-wetting occurs. By contrast, the grass beyond the tree has only a shallow (50cm) and transient drying effect. The effect of grass on the shallow drying of soil can be considerable, however, as shown by Insley (1982a) and Davies (1985). Biddle (1985) also demonstrated that the seasonal soil moisture profile under trees varies according to the soil type, as might be expected when rooting patterns and permeability are considered. Poplar and Oak were found to produce significantly greater effects than the other species investigated.

Annual plants such as agricultural cereals can also extract water from considerable depth in the soil. Durrant et al (1973) reported that barley sown in the spring in deep agricultural soil produced roots extending to below 1 metre depth by the end of June and was removing water at this depth. Evaporation from this soil would not affect the water content below about 0.3m depth.

Transpiration by vegetation is a strongly seasonal phenomenon, which in temperate European zones is out of phase with the rainfall and soil moisture cycle. As a result, the dormant season (winter) transpiration characteristics of the vegetation and the 'carry-over' effect of summer soil drying on subsequent winter soil moisture, are particularly important. This aspect is discussed by Coppin and Richards (1990) together with standard equations for the calculation of potential and actual evapo-transpiration by vegetation. They reported measurements showing that under young oak stands, winter soil moisture contents reached 16–20% in the top 600mm, whereas under comparable pine stands, soil moisture reached only 12–16% at the same time. Gray (1978) posed the crucial question: 'Does slope vegetation attenuate pore pressures or limit the rise in piezometric levels during a major and prolonged rainstorm sufficiently to make any difference?' None of the literature reviewed here provides a clear answer, demonstrating the need for further practical research.

A1.4.3   Increasing shear strength

Plant roots growing through a plane of potential failure increase the shear resistance by increasing the confining stress on the failure plane at the onset of shear. Coppin and Richards (1990) reviewed the work of various authors and presented a simplified model for the contribution of root tensile strength. They reported typical values for some vegetative components of the equation such as root density and tensile strength, and gave examples (from the literature) of the typical values for increases in soil cohesion due to roots. They stressed, however, that since the component values show great variability in natural vegetation, the model and data are not yet ready for use in the design of slopes.

The roots of herbaceous plants may be as valuable as those of woody plants in this mechanism of strengthening, since only roots below 15–20mm diameter contribute significantly to increased shear strength (Coppin and Richards, 1990). Experimental measurements of shear strength on soils with and without roots performed by Waldron, Endo and Tsuruta and others were reported by Gray (1978). Endo and Tsuruta found that percentage increase in shear strength due to young alder roots varied with root density and the contribution from normal stress, but for normal stress equivalent to approximately 2m of overburden, an increase in shear strength of up to 30% was provided by roots. Roots were particularly important where low normal stress applies, (i.e. at shallow depths).

Waldron and Dakessian (1982) made direct shear strength measurements in columns of soil in which various plants had been grown. They adjusted the matric potential to zero to remove the effect of soil moisture in a homogeneous saturated clay loam. Grasses, 6 months after sowing, doubled the shear resistance at 30cm depth. Three-year-old oak roots also doubled the shear resistance and 1-year-old alfalfa roots produced 4 times the resistance of unrooted soil. In columns where clay was placed over a dense sandy gravel, at 45cm depth, yellow pine roots produced a 50% increase in shear resistance at the interface after 16 months' growth, and a 150% increase after 52 months' growth. Seasonal growth patterns also apply to this mechanism since most herbaceous plants renew part of the root system each year. The effective root mass is reduced during each winter.

A1.4.4 Buttressing and soil arching

Roots of 20mm diameter or above are generally regarded as individual soil anchors in studies of slope strengthening. The tap roots and sinker roots of many trees penetrate into the deeper soil layers and anchor them against downslope movement. This produces:

a) a column of soil anchored by roots to the deep soil layers

b) a mass of soil above the tree, buttressed by a)

c) a zone of arching between adjacent buttressed masses (Coppin and Richards, 1990)

Many of the examples of this mechanism described by Gray (1978) relate to mature forest on cohesionless soils over fissured bedrock. Gray (1978) related these examples to mathematical equations for the effect of piles, and subsequently showed that even small increases in soil cohesion increased the stabilising effect of the fixed columns or 'root cylinders' considerably (reported in Coppin and Richards 1990). It appears, therefore, that this mechanism could play a substantial part in stabilising shallow failures once a column of anchorage to greater depth can be produced.

A1.4.5 Shading the surface

Prolonged extraction of moisture from plastic soils by plant roots or full sun can lead to deep cracking (Coppin and Richards 1990). These authors reported Anderson et al (1982) who surveyed a 1 in 2.5 clay motorway embankment of the M4. Few cracks were found on areas with dense grass cover, but poorly vegetated clay areas with exposed clay had extensive, deep cracking. These open cracks allowed winter rainfall to enter the slope and positive pore water pressure to develop leading to shallow seated failure.

Coppin and Richards argued that a vegetation cover would shade the surface from baking by the sun, and provide a root network which would restrain cracks from severe opening.

A1.4.6 Bio-engineering techniques for slope stabilisation

Living plant material has been used on its own, or combined with geotextiles, timber or other inert materials, to stabilise eroding slopes or slopes of loose material. These techniques have been proposed or described by many authors, including Gray (1978), Schiecht (1980) and Bache and MacAskill (1984). A comprehensive review was presented by Coppin and Richards (1990).

Composite construction using geotextiles and plant material is particularly suited to constructed embankments where the geotextile can be incorporated deeply. This technique has been used for the repair of failed existing slopes (Johnson, 1985) but cannot directly be applied to cuttings without over-excavation and reconstruction.

Brush-layering, in which live branches of willow or other easily rooted species are laid at 10–20° to the horizontal as a slope is built, is also applicable to embankment and to slope repair, but has typically been limited to less than 1m depth within the slope. Retaining walls, formed from gabions, anchored tyres, concrete or timber crib systems, can also include woody vegetation to bind the soil and improve the aesthetic appearance of the wall and create a long-term stabilising effect.

A1.5   SPECIES SELECTION FOR STABILISING VEGETATION

A1.5.1   Characteristics required

In Section A1.4, it was shown that vegetation could aid stabilisation by reducing soil moisture contents, rooting across the potential failure plane, and buttressing by anchoring columns of soil. To perform these functions, the vegetation will ideally require particular characteristics:

soil moisture:	rapid transpiration, winter transpiration activity, extensive root system
strengthening failure plane:	rapid, deep root growth (1.5m minimum), perennial root system
buttressing:	multiple deep 'sinker' roots with laterals
surface shading:	a high leaf-area ratio, persistence through hot summer periods.

In addition, the above-ground vegetation must not create an excessive maintenance burden or conflict with highway safety, and should provide a rapid initial cover to stabilise the topsoil layer. The vegetation should be regarded as a system, in which various components combine to provide the range of characteristics needed.

A1.5.2   Species characteristics

Many references describe the characteristics of particular species, but these references are not necessarily based on practical experience in a situation directly related to the site or problem under consideration. As plants may perform differently under different conditions, an assessment based on related examples or practical experience is required. Coppin and Richards (1990) produced lists of plants identified for particular bio-engineering functions, noting characteristic attributes of requirements.

A1.5.3   Effects of establishment method

The long-term behaviour of some species can be modified at an early stage of growth by cultural practices. It is therefore important that the function and necessary plant characteristics are clearly identified before establishment.

Possibly the most critical example of this is the effect of production methods on the deep-rooting ability of a tap-rooted species such as oak. Typical nursery production involves undercutting or transplanting at 1 or 2 years old to ensure a fibrous, compact root system capable of transplanting to the permanent site. This process removes the potential for the growth of a single deep 'tap' root. Container growing will also prevent tap rooting if the root system becomes cramped and twisted. The production of small seedlings in deep tube-shaped 'root-trainers' will allow the establishment of a tap-rooted tree. The effects of exposure of bare-root trees to root drying, even for short periods of a minute, have been clearly researched and reported (Insley 1980, for example) and yet many planting schemes fail or struggle to survive because of poor plant handling. Where the rapid growth of vegetation is an essential component of the construction process, this stage must receive the most rigorous control of workmanship.

Brush-layered vegetation will not grow tap roots but the technique is considered capable of producing deeply growing roots on steep slopes where the water table can be induced to retreat from the surface by plant evapo-transpiration and/or seasonal movement in ground water.

A1.5.4   Effects of vegetation management

The need for active management during the plant establishment phase, including fertilising, weed control around trees and shrubs, control of plant density where direct seeding has been used, and similar operation, is well covered in standard texts on plant establishment.

Management operations specific to the objectives set out for slope stabilisation will include:

- encouraging deep rooting
- maximising the transpiration from the canopy
- ensuring an adequate supply of nutrients
- avoiding the risk of wind throw or excessive surcharging.

These aspects were discussed by Coppin and Richards (1990). Deep rooting can be encouraged by the placing of initial fertilisers below the root zone of new plants, and by avoiding a moist nutrient-rich surface soil layer.

A1.6   MEASUREMENT AND MONITORING

A1.6.1   Parameters

The understanding of slope failure and the performance of various vegetation types in field trial conditions would be greatly increased by the collection of data on soil parameters at various depths throughout the trial. In-situ testing or monitoring will provide a more satisfactory data base than the testing of disturbed samples, with no damage to the vegetation.

The contribution of vegetation to maintaining low or negative pore water pressures can only reliably be monitored by direct measurement of this parameter at depths from the near-surface to well below the potential failure plane. Regular monitoring will identify whether re-wetting progresses from the surface downwards (external) or from groundwater laterally/upwards (internal), and will allow the magnitude of vegetation effects to be monitored as the vegetation develops.

Rainfall, and its effect on soil moisture, should be recorded to assist in the understanding of seasonal effects and vegetation effects. Soil strength measurements in the field would allow the progressive loss of strength, which occurs with re-wetting, to be monitored. Measurement of the appropriate strength parameters in the field or laboratory is not easy because the clay at construction does not reflect the properties found at the time of failure (Greenwood et al, 1985).

A1.6.2   Measurement methods

Pore water pressures were monitored by Crabb and West (1985) on an existing road embankment on the A45 near sections which had recently failed. Pore water pressure was monitored by an array of hydraulic piezometers, while a rain gauge recorded the rainfall. Both sets of instruments were logged automatically. Crabb and Atkinson (1991) further discussed field and laboratory testing methods in a paper on the analysis of slope failures. They used routine and special low-stress triaxial tests on tubed and reconstituted samples to determine the peak and critical strengths of the soils. Soil moisture can also be measured non-destructively using moisture block (electrical resistivity) or neutron probe devices. These methods were used in experiments on vegetation establishment by Insley (1982b) and Eason et al (1992), and by Biddle (1985) in soil moisture work described earlier. Greenwood et al (1985) reviewed possible methods to measure the strength of softened soils. Remoulded laboratory samples with increased moisture contents were considered unrepresentative of the field clay structure. Triaxial apparatus is, unless modified, unsuitable for the very low stress conditions of re-wetted field soils. Shear box tests were considered suitable for some situations, but this method requires destructive preparation and is not applicable to deeper layers. These authors concluded that until reliable methods can be developed, engineers must rely on back analysis of failed slopes, and interpretations based on indirect measurement.

Maximising transpiration requires the production of a large leaf area in an arrangement which avoids the creation of a zone of still, humid air around the leaves, and allows light to reach all the layers of vegetation. Coppicing species such as willow will produce a dense structure of upright branches, allowing light and wind penetration. Nutrients could be applied to the surface as fertilisers, but this may encourage root proliferation in the shallow soil layers. The inclusion of legumes in the vegetation will ensure that nitrogen is supplied within the root zone.

Where windthrow or excessive surcharge are judged to present unacceptable risks, the use of coppicing can create the desired density of vegetation as an even, relatively low canopy. The maximum acceptable height of individual trees or shrubs will determine the frequency of cutting required. As a continuity of the transpiration effect is essential for the slope stabilisation mechanism described in Section 4, coppicing should be carried out on a rotation, so that large temporarily bare areas are avoided.

A1.7   RELATED TRIAL WORK

A1.7.1   Introduction

As described in Section 1, (Introduction), there has been a considerable interest in trial work on erosion control and shallow stabilisation by vegetation and geotextiles, but very little work on the use of vegetation to control shallow failures in slopes.

Investigations of the modes of failure, causes and engineering solutions have been described in Sections 2 and 3 of this review.

A1.7.2   Related research

Research carried out for the Welsh Office by Richards, Moorehead and Laing between 1985 and 1990 was designed to evaluate the problem of surface instability in rock and scree slopes on road cuttings. It included site surveys, a literature review, and field trials (Richards, Moorehead and Laing, 1985–90), but was not directly related to the problem of shallow failure in over-consolidated clays.

Many other trials of hydraulic seeding, geotextile mats, seeded geotextiles and similar vegetation establishment methods have been reported (e.g., Rickson, 1992; Palmer, 1992).

A1.7.3 The need for further trials

The lack of practical research on techniques for the stabilisation of clay slopes prone to shallow failure can be seen both from the extent of the problem and the lack of trials experience. Particular aspects worthy of study are considered to be:

- the modification of soil moisture regimes by various types of vegetation, including herbaceous ground cover, shrubs and trees

- methods and species capable of rooting through the potential failure plane to strengthen this soil horizon, before soil re-wetting reaches critical limits

- the value of geotextiles, particularly in constructed embankments, as deeply buried 'envelopes' to restrain softened soils.

A trial set up in an area known to be prone to slope failure could provide valuable data of use in future slope design, and act as a demonstration of the validity of bio-engineering techniques for such applications.

A1.8 LITERATURE REVIEW REFERENCES

ANDERSON, M.G., HUBBERD, M.G. and KNEALE, P.E. (1982)
The influence of shrinkage cracks on pore water pressures within a clay embankment.
Quarterly Journal of Engineering Geology, 15 (1) 9–14 (reported in Coppin and Richards, 1990).

ANDERSON, M.G. and KNEALE, P.E. (1980)
Pore water pressure changes in a road embankment. *Journal of the Institution of Highway Engineers*, May 1980, 11-17.

BACHE, D.H. and MACASKILL, I.A. (1984)
Vegetation in Civil and Landscape Engineering
Granada Publishing, London.

BARKER, D.H. (1986)
Biodegradable geotextiles for erosion control and slope stabilisation. *Civil Engineering*, June 1986, 13–15.

BARKER, D.H. (1991)
Slope stabilisation by vertical soil reinforcement.
In. *Proceedings ICE conference, 'Slope Stability Engineering'*. Paper 47

BIDDLE, P.G. (1985)
Trees and buildings.
In. *Advances in Practical Arboriculture* (symposium)
Published as *Bulletin 65*, Forestry Commission 1987
121–131.

BRITISH STANDARDS INSTITUTION (1981)
Code of Practice for Earth Works, BS6031

COPPIN, N.J. and RICHARDS, I.G. (1990)
Use of vegetation in civil engineering
CIRIA Book 10, London.

CRABB, G.I. and ATKINSON, J.H. (1991)
Determination of soil strength parameters for the analysis of highway slope failures. In proceedings ICE Conference, 'Slope Stability Engineering'.
Paper 2

CRABB, G.I. and WEST, G. (1985)
Monitoring pore water pressures in an embankment. In *Proceedings of Symposium on Failures in Earthworks Institution of Civil Engineers* (London), Technical Note 4.

CUTLER, D.G. and RICHARDSON, I.B.K. (1989)
Tree roots and Buildings (2nd edn), Longman Scientific and Technical, London.

DAVIES, R.J. (1985)
Weed competition and broadleaved tree establishment.
In. *Advances in Practical Arboriculture* (symposium), published as *Bulletin 65*
Forestry Commission 1987, 91–9,

DEPARTMENT OF THE ENVIRONMENT (1991)
Handbook on the Design of Tips and Related Structures.
HMSO.

DURRANT, M.J., COVE, B.J.G., MESSEM, A.B. and DRAYCOTT, A.P. (1973)
Growth of crop roots in relation to soil moisture extraction. *Annals of Applied Biology* 74, 387–94.

EASON, W.R., TOMLINSON, H.F. and HAINSWORTH, C. (1992)
Effect of ground vegetation on root distribution of ash trees. In. Vegetation management in forestry, amenity and conservation areas. *Aspects of Applied Botany*, 29, 225–231, Association of Applied Biologists.

FARRAR, D.M. (1978)
Settlement and pore water pressure dissipation within an embankment built of London Clay, In. *Clay Fills*, Institution of Civil Engineers, London 101–106.

FARRAR, D.M. (1984)
Long term changes in pore water pressure within an embankment built of London Clay TRRL Report.

GARRETT, E. and WALE, J.H. (1985)
Performance of embankments and cuttings in Gault Clay in Kent. In: *Proceedings of Symposium on Failures in Earthworks*. Institution of Civil Engineers, London, Paper 7.

GRAY, D.H. (1978)
Role of woody vegetation in reinforcing soils and stabilising slopes. In: *Symposium on Soil reinforcing and Stabilising Techniques.* New South Wales Institute of Technology 1978, 253–306

GREENWOOD, J.R., HOLT, D.A. and HERRICK, G.W. (1985)
Shallow slips in highway embankments constructed of over-consolidated clay. In: Proceedings of Symposium on Failures in Earthworks, Institution of Civil Engineers, London, Paper 6.

INSLEY, H. (1980)
Moving plants safely.
In Research for practical arboriculture (seminar), Forestry Commission 1980
49–57

INSLEY, H. (1982a)
The influence of post planting maintenance on the growth of newly planted broadleaved
trees. In *Conference on Cost Effective Amenity Landscape Management* HEA 1982
74–80

INSLEY, H. (1982b)
The effects of stock type, handling and sward control on amenity tree establishment.
Unpublished PhD Thesis, Wye College, University of London

JOHNSON, P.E. (1985)
Maintenance and repair of highway embankments: studies of seven methods of
treatment. TRRL Research Report 30.

PALMER, J.P. (1992)
The use of biodegradable geofabrics to control highway slope erosion. In Proceedings
UK *Coir Geotextile Seminar Coir Board of India.*

PARSONS, A.W. and PERRY, J. (1985)
Slope stability problems in ageing highway earthworks.
In: Proceedings of symposium on failures in earth-works.
Institution of Civil Engineers (London) paper 5

RICHARDS, MOOREHEAD and LAING (1985–90)
Stabilisation and revegetation of rock and scree slopes on road cuttings. Literature
review. Assessment of revegetation trials. Erosion control trials. Site classification as the
basis for the design, management and repair of vegetation on highway margins.
Unpublished reports to the Welsh Office.

RICKSON, J. (1992)
Soil erosion processes and their control. In proceedings UK *Coir Geotextile Seminar*
Coir Board of India.

SCHIECHTL, H.M. (1980)
Bioengineering for Land Reclamation and Conservation
University of Alberta Press, Edmonton.

WALDRON, L.J. and DAKESSIAN, S. (1982)
Effect of grass, legume and tree roots on soil shearing resistance. Soil Science Society
of America Journal, 46 (5), 894–99.

Appendix A2 Specification for trial areas

The actual contract documents used were based upon the following specification. Amendments made to the specification are shaded.

A2.1   CULTIVATION

A2.1.1   Areas A, B, C

All areas will be cultivated to a minimum depth of 150mm leaving this layer free from compaction. For seeded treatment (i.e. 2,5,6) a fine surface tilth will be created suitable for the sowing of grass seed.

Change to specification	Cultivation: Areas A, B, C Spring tine cultivated to a depth of 225mm and rotovated to a 150mm depth.

A2.1.2   Areas D, E

On these areas either shallow (D) or no topsoil (E) has been placed. Cultivation will therefore be to the depth of the placed topsoils, approximately 50mm, on soiled areas and to a minimum of 50mm on areas E. A fine surface tilth will be created on all treatment to be seeded.

A2.2   FERTILISER

Four fertiliser regimes are defined for the trial site based on the soil analysis and treatment requirement. The regimes are, or are equivalent to:

i   =   5:20:20 compound at 40g/m2 plus 0:22:0 superphosphate at 25g/m2

ii   =   0:20:20 compound at 40g/m2 plus 0:22:0 superphosphate at 25g/m2

iii   =   10:20:20 compound at 80g/m2

iv   =   No fertiliser to be applied

Changes to specification	Regime i: 10:20:20 compound fertiliser in lieu of specified.
	Regime ii: 0:20:30 compound fertiliser in lieu of specified.

Plot treatments are shown in Table 4.1 of the main report.

A2.3 WEED CONTROL

If weed growth has developed on any areas prior to planting/sowing this shall be sprayed off with a contact herbicide applied to the manufacturers recommendations.

A2.4 PLANTING SPECIFICATION

A2.4.1 Treatment 1: willow and alder

Species	% Composition
Alnus glutinosa (Common alder)	20
Salix caprea (Goat willow)	20
S. cinerea (Grey sallow)	20
S. purpurea (Purple osier)	20
S. viminalis (Common osier)	20
Total number of plants required	750

Planting operations

Alnus glutinosa shall be bare root stock, one-year transplants, and salix one-year rooted cuttings. All stock to be notch planted at lm centres, staggered. After planting, each plant to be cut just above a bud at approximately 200mm above ground level. Planting will be random across the plots.

Treatment 1: Willow and Alder (a, b, c, d, e) – Page 2 Seed mix of European provenance accepted.

A2.4.2 Treatment 2: Shrubs – broom and gorse mix

Species	% Composition
Cytisus scoparius (Common broom)	20
Hippophae rhamnoides (Sea buckthorn)	20
Lupinus arboreus (Tree lupin)	20
L. polyphyllos (Perennial blue lupin)	20
Ulex europaeus (European Gorse)	20
Total quantity of seed required	2.25kg

Seeding

Prior to sowing, the seeds shall be thoroughly scarified (by abrasion), and mixed well to form a random composition. Each plot shall be divided into four equal portions and each sown separately to ensure an even spread. Prior to sowing the mixed seed shall be blended with dry sand or sawdust, to 'bulk up' by 3 times. Sowing shall be by hand at a rate of 3.0g/m2. Following sowing, the seed shall be carefully raked into the surface of the soil to cover the seed.

Timing

Seed shall be sown in March.

A2.4.3   Treatment 3: bramble mix

Species	% Composition
Rosa canina (Dog rose)	25
R. pimpinellifolia (Shrub rose variety)	15
Rubus fruticosus (Bramble)	35
R. tricolor (Ornamental bramble)	25
Total number of plant required	530

Planting operations

All plants shall be bare root stock, one-year transplants, notch planted randomly at 750mm centres in staggered rows. Stock should be planted in a random mix with single species groups not exceeding 5 plants. If only container stock is available then 1.0 litre pots shall be used.

A2.4.4   Treatment 4: Shrubs – evergreen groundcover mix

Species	% Composition
Cotoneaster dammeri (Cotoneaster variety)	50
Prunus laurocerasus 'Zabeliana' (Laurel variety)	25
Vinca minor (Lesser periwinkle)	25
Total number of plants required	830

Planting operations

Plants shall be open ground stock if possible, one year transplants, randomly notch planted at 600mm centres in staggered rows. If only container-grown stock is available, 1.0-litre pots shall be used.

A2.4.5   Treatment 5: forbs and grass

Species	% Composition
Forbs (Herbs)	
Achillea millefolium (yarrow)	4
Anthyllis vulnerana (Kidney vetch)	2
Centaurea nigra (Black knapweed)	4
Chrysanthemum leucanthemum (Oxeye daisy)	4
Lotus corniculatus (Birdsfoot trefoil)	4
Hypericum perforatum (Common St.Johns wort)	2
Medicago lupilina (Black medic)	2
Knautia arvensis (Field scabious)	4
Plantago lanceolata (Ribwort plantain)	2
Silene alba (White campion)	2

Grasses

Agrostis tenuis (A. capillaris) (Common bent)	10
Alopecurus pratensis (Common foxtail)	5
Festuca longifolia (Hard fescue)	10
F. rubra litoralis (Slender creeping red fescue)	20
F. rubra rubra (Creeping red fescue)	20
Holcus lanatus (Yorkshire fog)	5
Total quantity of seed required	4.5kg

Seeding

Prior to sowing the seeds shall be thoroughly and evenly mixed together, and blended with dry sand or sawdust, to 'bulk up' the seed by 3 times. Each plot shall be divided into four equal portions and each sown separately to ensure an even spread. Sowing shall be by hand to give an even distribution of 6.0g/m2 over the site. Following sowing the seed shall be lightly raked into the surface of soil to cover the seed.

Timing

Sowing shall take place in March.

A2.4.6 Treatment 6: DTp grass mix

Species	% Composition
Dwarf perennial rye grass	20
Creeping bent	2.5
Highland browntop	7.5
Sheeps fescue	15
Slenda creeping red fescue	25
Strong creeping red fescue	25
Wild white clover 'Pertina'	5
Total quantity of seed required	1.8kg

Seeding

As for Treatment No. 5 (forbs and grasses).

A2.4.7 Treatment 7: bare ground

This area is to be left bare throughout the trial – no fertilising, planting or seeding are to be undertaken.

To maintain bare ground in these plots, an approved herbicide, such as glyphosate, shall be applied twice yearly, in April and September, at the manufacturers recommended rates.

A2.5   MAINTENANCE

A2.5.1   General specification

Maintenance period

It is envisaged that the trial plots will be managed in the long term. However, for the purposes of this Contract, maintenance will be undertaken for a period of 3 years following certification of planting and seeding operations.

Replacement of failures

Any plants which die or fail to thrive or seeded areas which fail within the first 12 months of maintenance as a result of any cause within the control of the Contractor, shall be replaced in accordance with the specification at the Contractors own expense in the first available planting season. The Supervising Officer shall inspect the site with the Contractor during the first 12 months of maintenance to agree losses.

Re-firming after frost

During the first year of maintenance, the ground shall be re-firmed around plants after periods of frost, wind or excessive surface runoff. Such firming shall be done by treading the soil around the roots and root collar with the heel of the foot.

Weed control

During the first year of maintenance weeds shall be controlled by herbicide application or hand-weeding around the base of each plant, and by spot treatment within the grass and wildflower swards. Each plot shall be maintained in a weed-free condition by maintenance operations in April, July and September. Weeds shall be removed off site from the 'forbs and grass' plots (Treatment 5).

During years 2 and 3 of maintenance, weed control shall be undertaken in April of each year, and additionally, if necessary, to remove particularly invasive and pernicious weeds.

Day rate

Allocation of time to specific maintenance requirements on the plot trials is not practical. Therefore day rate costs should be included on the basis of:
- Year 1 5 days
- Year 2 5 days
- Year 3 10 days

Actual site maintenance works will be specified following site inspections.

A2.5.2   Treatment 1: willow and alder

Willow coppice regime

In addition to the cut required at the time of planting, as specified in Section 4.1, all willows and alders will be coppiced in the third year of planting. Coppicing shall be undertaken at a height of 200mm above ground level. There should be a neat cut, leaving a sloping face, and ensuring that no torn or ragged ends are produced. All cut material shall be removed off site.

Fertiliser application

Area E shall be treated with 20g/m2 of 5:25:20 compound fertiliser in the second maintenance year to retain fertility.

A2.5.3   Treatment 2: Shrubs – broom and gorse mix

Vegetation management

Visits will be required for the purpose of pruning, thinning and removing shrubs as directed by the Supervising Officer. Such operations are unlikely to be required in the first year of maintenance. Any cutting and pruning shall be undertaken to leave neat, sloping cuts. Any removal of shrubs shall mean cutting to ground level, and the removal of the sub-aerial portion of the plant, which should be taken off-site, leaving the roots in the ground.

Fertiliser application

As for Treatment 1.

A2.5.4   Treatment 3: Shrubs – bramble mix

Vegetation management

As for Treatment 2.

Fertiliser application

As for Treatment 1.

A2.5.5   Treatment 4: Shrubs – evergreen groundcover mix

Vegetation management

As for Treatment 2.

Fertiliser application

As for Treatment 1.

A2.5.6   Treatment 5: forbs and grass

Cutting regime

Plots with treatment 5 shall be mown once annually in late September to a height above ground level of 100mm. Cuttings shall be removed off site.

A2.5.7   **Treatment 6: DTp grass mix**

Cutting regime

Plots with treatment 6 shall be mown three times in the first year of maintenance to leave a nominal 50mm after the first cut and 75mm after the second and third cuts. The first cut shall be carried out when the grass has reached 100mm, the second and third at 125mm. In subsequent years, the plots shall be mown twice annually in April and August to a height of 75mm.

Fertiliser application

As for Treatment 1.

Plates

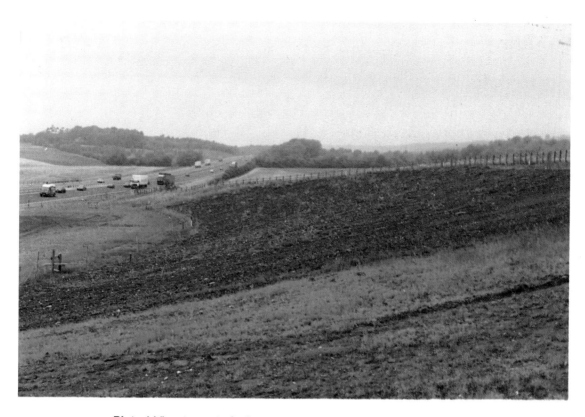

Plate 1 View to west of primary site (May 1994)

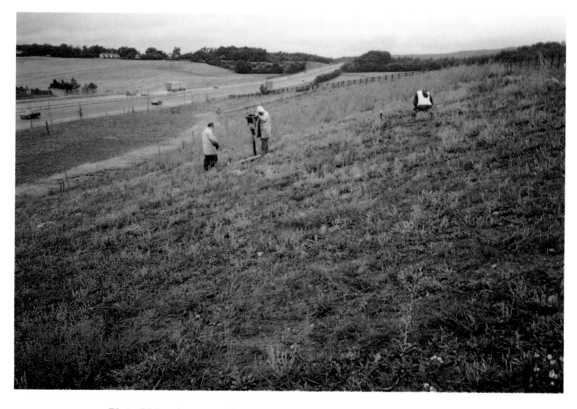

Plate 2 View to west with geodrive sampling (September 1994)

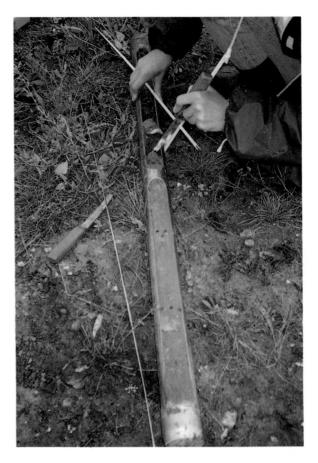

Plate 3 Geodrive tube and root growth count (September 1994)

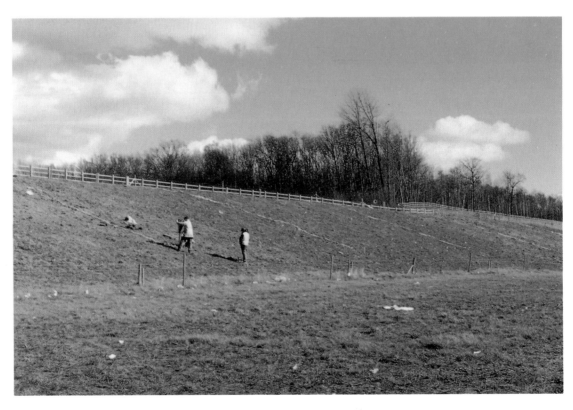

Plate 4 Geodrive sampling (March 1995)

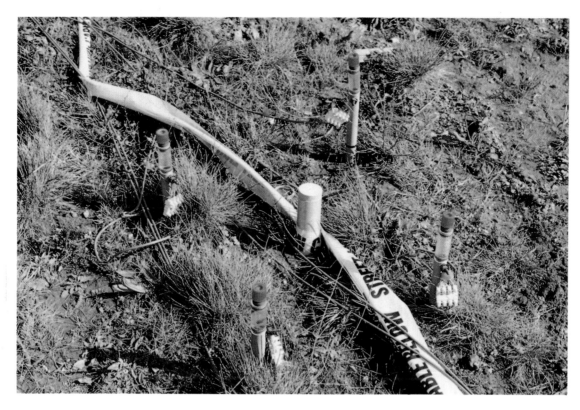

Plate 5 Instrumentation cluster (March 1995)

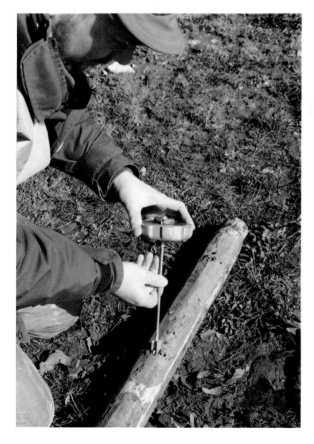

Plate 6 Hand vane testing (March 1995)

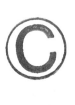